INTERMITTENT FASTING 101 FOR WOMEN OVER 40

Revitalize Your Energy And Health:The A-Z and No fuss guide for beginners and busy women.

Ava T. Hills

TABLE OF CONTENTS

CHAPTER 5

OVERCOMING COMMON CHALLENGES

CHAPTER 6

INTERMITTENT FASTING AND HORMONAL HEALTH

CHAPTER 7

TIPS FOR BUSY WOMEN

INTRODUCTION

If you're holding this book, you're probably a woman over 40, like me, looking for a way to boost your energy, improve your health, and reclaim your vitality without all the fuss and complexity and let me tell you, I get it.

Like many of you, I found myself feeling exhausted, sluggish, and out of shape as I entered my 40s. Juggling the demands of work, family, and personal responsibilities left little time for self-care, and I struggled to find a sustainable way to prioritize my health.

It was during one particularly challenging period that I stumbled upon intermittent fasting. Frustrated by my lack of energy and persistent weight gain, I began researching different approaches to wellness. That's when I came across the concept of intermittent fasting—a simple yet powerful strategy that promised to revitalize both body and mind.

At first, I was skeptical. Like many of you, I had been conditioned to believe that constant grazing and strict dietary restrictions were the keys to weight loss and overall health. The idea of voluntarily abstaining from food for extended periods seemed counterintuitive, if not downright risky. But as I delved deeper into the science behind intermittent fasting and heard countless success stories from women just like me, I became intrigued. From improving metabolic health to reducing inflammation, intermittent fasting offered a myriad of benefits that promised to revolutionize my health and wellness. Could this be the answer I was looking for? I thought I had everything to gain and nothing to lose, so I gave it a shot.

What started as a simple experiment soon turned into a life-changing discovery. The results were nothing short of transformative. Within weeks of adopting an intermittent fasting routine, I noticed a dramatic increase in my energy levels, mental clarity, and overall sense of well-being. The stubborn pounds that had plagued me for years began to melt away, and I found myself feeling more confident and empowered than ever before. But perhaps the most remarkable aspect of my journey was how effortless it felt. Unlike restrictive diets that left me feeling deprived and frustrated, intermittent fasting allowed me to enjoy the foods I loved while still achieving my health and fitness goals. It was a revelation—a sustainable lifestyle change that I could maintain for the long haul.

Inspired by my own experience, I set out to share the transformative power of intermittent fasting with women everywhere. In this book, I've distilled everything I've learned along the way into a comprehensive guide that's tailored specifically for women over 40. Intermittent fasting is not just about losing weight or fitting into a smaller dress size – it's about reclaiming our health so that we can live our lives to the fullest. It's about saying goodbye to crash diets and endless cycles of restriction and deprivation, and hello to a sustainable way of eating that nourishes both body and soul.

So, if you're ready to embark on this journey with me, I invite you to dive into the pages of this book and discover the wonders of intermittent fasting for yourself.

From the basics of intermittent fasting to practical tips for incorporating it into your busy lifestyle, you'll find everything you need to embark on your own journey to renewed vitality and health. Whether you're looking to shed excess weight, boost your energy levels, or simply feel better in your own skin, intermittent fasting can help you achieve your goals. this book is your comprehensive guide to reinvigorating and reclaiming your health – one fasting window at a time.

Together, let's unlock the secrets of intermittent fasting and embark on a journey towards a happier, healthier, and more vibrant version of ourselves. Are you ready to join me?

Let's dive in!

CHAPTER 1

UNDERSTANDING INTERMITTENT FASTING

What is Intermittent Fasting?

Intermittent fasting is a dietary approach that focuses on when you eat rather than what you eat. It involves alternating periods of fasting with periods of eating, and it has gained popularity for its potential health benefits, including weight loss, improved metabolic health, and increased longevity. But how exactly does intermittent fasting work?

Understanding the Basics of Intermittent Fasting

At its core, intermittent fasting is a dietary pattern that involves cycling between periods of fasting and eating. Unlike traditional calorie-restriction diets, which focus on what you eat, intermittent fasting focuses on when you eat. By alternating between fasting periods and eating windows, intermittent fasting aims to optimize the body's metabolic processes and promote various health benefits. Despite its potential benefits, intermittent fasting may not be suitable for everyone. Pregnant or breastfeeding women, individuals with a history of eating disorders, and those with certain medical conditions should consult with a healthcare professional before starting an intermittent fasting regimen.

The Science Behind It

When you consume food, especially carbohydrates, your body breaks it down into glucose, which serves as the primary Source of energy. Extra glucose is converted to glycogen in the muscles and liver for later usage. Between meals, when glucose levels drop, the body taps into these glycogen stores to maintain energy levels.

During a fast, however, when you abstain from consuming calories for a certain period, the body depletes its glycogen reserves and begins to rely on alternative sources of energy, such as fat stores.

This metabolic shift triggers a series of physiological changes in the body that contribute to the health benefits of intermittent fasting. These changes include:

- **Ketosis: The Key to Fat Burning**

One of the hallmark features of intermittent fasting is the induction of ketosis, a metabolic state in which the body produces ketone bodies from fat stores to fuel cellular energy needs. Ketosis typically occurs after an extended period of fasting, usually around 12-24 hours, depending on individual factors such as metabolism and activity level. During ketosis, the liver converts fatty acids into ketone bodies, which can cross the blood-brain barrier and provide energy to the brain. This process not only facilitates fat burning but also helps preserve lean muscle mass, making intermittent fasting an effective strategy for weight loss and body composition improvement.

- **Hormone Regulation**

Intermittent fasting also exerts profound effects on hormone regulation, influencing key hormones involved in appetite control, metabolism, and energy balance. Some of the key hormones affected by intermittent fasting include:

Insulin: Fasting lowers insulin levels, which promotes fat burning and enhances insulin sensitivity, reducing the risk of insulin resistance and type 2 diabetes.

Growth Hormone: Fasting increases the secretion of growth hormone, which stimulates fat breakdown and muscle growth, contributing to improved body composition.

Norepinephrine: Fasting activates the sympathetic nervous system, leading to increased release of norepinephrine, a hormone that enhances fat mobilization and metabolic rate.By modulating these hormone levels, intermittent fasting helps optimize metabolic function and promote weight loss while preserving muscle mass and metabolic health.

- **Cellular Repair and Autophagy**

In addition to its effects on metabolism and hormone regulation, intermittent fasting also triggers cellular repair processes such as autophagy. Autophagy is a natural cellular detoxification mechanism in which damaged or dysfunctional cellular components are broken down and recycled to maintain cellular integrity.

During fasting, when energy reserves are low, the body upregulates autophagy to clear out cellular debris and promote cellular renewal. This process not only helps remove toxins and waste products but also supports overall cellular health and longevity.

Types of Intermittent Fasting

There are several different approaches to intermittent fasting, each with its own unique fasting and eating windows. Several often employed methods include:

- The 16/8 Method calls for restricting your eating window to 8 hours and fasting for 16 hours every day.. For example, you might skip breakfast and only eat between noon and 8 p.m.
- 5:2 Diet: With this approach, you eat normally for five days of the week and then restrict your calorie intake to 500-600 calories per day for the remaining two days.
- Alternate-Day Fasting: As the name suggests, this method involves fasting every other day, either by consuming no calories or significantly reducing calorie intake.
- Eat-Stop-Eat: Using this method, you fast for a whole day once or twice a week, during which you don't eat anything.

- The Warrior Diet: This method involves fasting for 20 hours each day and consuming all your calories within a 4-hour eating window in the evening.

Regardless of the specific approach, the goal of intermittent fasting is to create a calorie deficit by reducing the number of hours spent eating, thereby promoting weight loss and other health benefits.

Benefits of Intermittent Fasting to women over forty

While intermittent fasting offers a wide range of benefits for individuals of all ages, women over 40 may particularly stand to gain from this dietary approach due to the following reasons:

1. Weight Management: Metabolism tends to slow down with age, making it more challenging for women over 40 to lose weight or maintain a healthy weight. Intermittent fasting can help overcome metabolic resistance by promoting fat burning and calorie restriction, making it easier to achieve weight loss goals.

2. Bone Health: Women are at increased risk of osteoporosis and bone loss as they age, especially after menopause. Intermittent fasting has been shown to support bone health by increasing the production of osteocalcin, a hormone that promotes bone formation and strength.

3. Heart Health: Cardiovascular disease is a leading cause of death among women over 40, with risk factors such as high blood pressure, cholesterol levels, and inflammation. Intermittent fasting can help improve cardiovascular health by lowering blood pressure, reducing cholesterol levels, and decreasing inflammation in the body.

4. Mental Well-being: Many women experience changes in mood and cognitive function during perimenopause and menopause, including symptoms such as anxiety, depression, and brain fog. Intermittent fasting may help improve mood and cognitive function by promoting the production of neurotransmitters such as serotonin and dopamine, which are essential for mood regulation and mental well-being.

5. Improved Metabolic Health: Intermittent fasting has been shown to improve various markers of metabolic health, including insulin sensitivity, blood sugar control, and cholesterol levels. By regulating hormone levels and enhancing metabolic function, intermittent fasting can help reduce the risk of chronic diseases such as type 2 diabetes and heart disease.

6. Brain Function: Fasting has been linked to cognitive benefits such as improved focus, mental clarity, and memory. By promoting the production of brain-derived neurotrophic factor (BDNF), a protein that supports neuronal growth and function, intermittent fasting may help protect against age-related cognitive decline and neurodegenerative diseases.

7. Increased Energy Levels: Many individuals report experiencing increased energy and

vitality during fasting periods, as the body shifts from relying on glucose for energy to burning fat. By tapping into fat stores for fuel, intermittent fasting can provide a steady source of energy throughout the day, reducing feelings of fatigue and lethargy.

8. Reduced Inflammation: Chronic inflammation is linked to a variety of health conditions, including autoimmune diseases, arthritis, and cardiovascular disease. Intermittent fasting has been shown to reduce markers of inflammation in the body, potentially lowering the risk of inflammatory diseases and promoting overall health and well-being.

9. Cellular Repair and Longevity: Fasting triggers autophagy, a cellular repair process in which damaged or dysfunctional cells are broken down and recycled. By promoting cellular renewal and rejuvenation, intermittent fasting may help delay the aging process and extend lifespan.

10. Hormonal Balance: Women experience significant hormonal changes as they age, particularly during perimenopause and menopause. Intermittent fasting can help stabilize hormone levels, reduce symptoms such as hot flashes and mood swings, and improve overall hormonal balance.

Demystifying Myths of Intermittent Fasting

Myths surrounding intermittent fasting are common and separating fact from fiction to help you make informed decisions about incorporating this dietary approach into your lifestyle.

Myth 1: Your Metabolism Is Slowed Down by Intermittent Fasting

One of the most persistent myths about intermittent fasting is that it slows down your metabolism, making it harder to lose weight and maintain a healthy weight. However, research suggests that intermittent fasting may actually have the opposite effect. By promoting fat burning and preserving lean muscle mass, intermittent fasting can help maintain metabolic rate and improve metabolic health over time.

Studies have shown that intermittent fasting can increase levels of norepinephrine, a hormone that boosts metabolic rate and enhances fat burning.

Myth 2: Intermittent Fasting Causes Muscle Loss

Another common concern about intermittent fasting is that it leads to muscle loss, particularly during fasting periods. While it's true that fasting can increase breakdown of muscle tissue for energy, this effect is generally minimal and can be mitigated by maintaining adequate protein intake and engaging in regular resistance training.

Research suggests that intermittent fasting may actually help preserve muscle mass while promoting fat loss. By stimulating growth hormone secretion and increasing protein synthesis, intermittent fasting supports muscle growth and repair, even during fasting periods.

Myth 3: Intermittent Fasting is Unsafe for Women

There's a misconception that intermittent fasting is unsafe or inappropriate for women, particularly those of reproductive age or going through menopause. However, research indicates that intermittent fasting can be safe and effective for women when done properly and tailored to individual needs.

Myth 4: Nutrient Deficiencies Result from Intermittent Fasting

Concerns have been raised about the potential for nutrient deficiencies on an intermittent fasting diet, particularly if fasting periods are prolonged or if there's a lack of variety in food choices. While it's true that fasting can reduce overall calorie intake and may require careful attention to nutrient balance, it's entirely possible to meet your nutritional needs while practicing intermittent fasting.

By focusing on nutrient-dense foods such as fruits, vegetables, lean proteins, and healthy fats during eating windows, you can ensure that you're getting essential vitamins, minerals, and micronutrients. Additionally, supplementation may be recommended for certain nutrients, especially if you have specific dietary restrictions or health concerns.

Myth 5: Intermittent Fasting is Only for Weight Loss

While weight loss is one of the most well-known benefits of intermittent fasting, it's not the only reason to consider this dietary approach. Intermittent fasting offers a wide range of potential health benefits beyond weight management, including improved metabolic health, increased energy levels, enhanced cognitive function, and even longevity.Many people find that intermittent fasting helps them feel more focused, energized, and mentally sharp, which can enhance productivity and overall well-being.

Whether you're looking to lose weight, improve insulin sensitivity, or enhance cognitive function, intermittent fasting offers a valuable tool for achieving your health and wellness goals. By approaching intermittent fasting with an open mind and a willingness to experiment, you can discover how this dietary approach can support your journey to optimal health.

CHAPTER 2
GETTING STARTED WITH INTERMITTENT FASTING

Assessing Your Current Health Status

Assessing your current health status is akin to taking stock of your resources before embarking on a journey. It provides invaluable insight into your body's strengths, weaknesses, and areas that may require special attention. When starting intermittent fasting, knowing your health status enables you to set realistic goals, identify potential challenges, and make informed decisions about your fasting protocols. This involves assessing various aspects of your physical, mental, and emotional well-being.

Here are some practical tips to help you evaluate your health baseline:

- **Consult with a Healthcare Professional**
Before making any significant changes to your diet or lifestyle, it's wise to consult with a healthcare professional. They can provide personalized guidance based on your individual health history, current conditions, and goals. Your healthcare provider may perform tests or evaluations to assess

your overall health and identify any potential risks or contraindications for intermittent fasting.

- **Evaluate Your Medical History**

Take some time to review your medical history, including any chronic conditions, past surgeries, or medications you're currently taking. Certain health conditions may require modifications to your fasting plan or close monitoring to ensure safety. Be sure to disclose any relevant information to your healthcare provider for personalized recommendations.

- **Assess Your Current Diet and Lifestyle**

Consider your current dietary habits and lifestyle factors that may impact your health. Are you consuming a balanced diet rich in whole foods, or do you rely heavily on processed or fast foods? Do you engage in regular physical activity, or is your lifestyle predominantly sedentary? Evaluating these factors can help you identify areas for improvement and set realistic goals for your intermittent fasting journey.

- **Measure Key Health Metrics**

Tracking key health metrics can provide valuable insights into your overall health and progress over time. Consider measuring metrics such as body weight, body mass index (BMI), waist circumference, blood pressure, blood glucose levels, and cholesterol levels. These measurements can serve as benchmarks to monitor your health throughout your intermittent fasting journey.

Practical Tips for Assessing Your Health

Now that you have a better understanding of what to consider when assessing your current health status, here are some practical tips to help you get started:

- Keep a Health Journal: Start a journal to track your dietary intake, physical activity, sleep patterns, mood, and any symptoms or changes in health. This journal can serve as a valuable tool for identifying patterns, tracking progress, and communicating with your healthcare provider.
- Schedule Regular Check-Ups: Make it a priority to schedule regular check-ups with your healthcare provider to monitor your health and discuss any concerns or questions you may have. These appointments allow for ongoing evaluation and adjustments to your intermittent fasting plan as needed.
- Listen to Your Body: Pay attention to how intermittent fasting affects your body. If you experience any adverse effects or symptoms, such as dizziness, fatigue, headaches, or mood changes, it's essential to listen to your body and adjust your fasting approach accordingly. Don't hesitate to seek guidance from a healthcare professional if needed.
- Monitor Progress: Continuously monitor your progress and reassess your health status periodically. Keep track of any changes in key health metrics, improvements in energy

levels, changes in body composition, and overall well-being. Celebrate your successes and make adjustments as necessary to stay on track towards your health goals.

Choosing the Right Intermittent Fasting Method

Now that you've assessed your current health status, it's time to explore the various intermittent fasting methods and choose the one that best suits you. Embarking on an intermittent fasting journey requires careful consideration of the various fasting methods available. Each method offers unique benefits and challenges, making it essential to choose one that aligns with your lifestyle, preferences, and health goals.

Understanding Different Intermittent Fasting Methods

Intermittent fasting encompasses a range of fasting schedules, each with its own unique approach to meal timing and fasting duration. Here are some popular intermittent fasting methods:

- 16/8 Method: Also known as the Leangains protocol, the 16/8 method involves fasting for 16 hours each day and restricting your eating window to 8 hours. For example, you might fast from 8:00 PM until 12:00 PM the next day, then eat your meals between 12:00 PM and 8:00 PM.
- 5:2 Diet: In the 5:2 diet, you eat normally for five days of the week and restrict your calorie intake to 500-600 calories on two

non-consecutive days. These fasting days can be spread throughout the week as desired.

- Eat-Stop-Eat: With this method, you fast for a day once or twice a week. For example, you might fast from dinner one day until dinner the next day, consuming no calories during the fasting period.
- Alternate-Day Fasting: Alternate-day fasting involves alternating between fasting days and non-fasting days. You take in minimal to no calories during fasting days, and you eat regularly when you're not fasting
- Warrior Diet: The Warrior Diet involves fasting for 20 hours each day and consuming all your calories within a 4-hour eating window, typically in the evening.

Practical Tips for Choosing the Right Intermittent Fasting Method

With numerous intermittent fasting methods available, selecting the right one can feel overwhelming. Here are some practical tips to help you choose the fasting method that best suits your needs:

1. Consider Your Lifestyle: Evaluate your daily routine, work schedule, and social commitments. Choose a fasting method that seamlessly integrates into your lifestyle without causing undue stress or disruption. For example: If you have a hectic work

schedule and prefer to eat larger meals in the evening, the Warrior Diet or 16/8 method may be more suitable, as they allow for a longer fasting window during the day.

2. Health Status and Goals: Take into account your current health status, any existing medical conditions and consult with your healthcare provider before starting intermittent fasting, especially if you have any underlying health concerns. For example: If you have diabetes, hypertension, or a history of eating disorders, it's essential to consult with a healthcare provider to determine the most appropriate fasting approach and monitor your health closely.

3. Assess Your Hunger Tolerance: Reflect on your relationship with hunger and your ability to tolerate fasting periods. Some people may find shorter fasting windows more manageable, while others may thrive with longer fasting durations. If you're new to fasting or have low hunger tolerance, starting with a shorter fasting window, such as 14/10 or 16/8, can help ease you into the practice gradually.

4. Set Realistic Goals: Clarify your health goals and expectations for intermittent fasting. Whether you're aiming to lose weight, improve metabolic health, or enhance mental clarity, choose a fasting method aligned with

your objectives. For example: If your primary goal is weight loss, you may opt for more aggressive fasting protocols, such as the 5:2 diet or alternate-day fasting, to create a larger calorie deficit. However, prioritize sustainable and healthy weight loss over rapid or extreme methods.

5. Listen to Your Body: Pay attention to how your body responds to different fasting methods. Experiment with various protocols and adjust as needed based on your energy levels, hunger cues, and overall well-being.

Exploring Trial and Error

Finding the right intermittent fasting method may require some trial and error. Don't be discouraged if you don't immediately find the perfect fit. Do not forget that there is no one-size-fits-all method for alternating periods of fasting. Embrace experimentation, listen to your body, and trust yourself to find the method that resonates with you. When I first started intermittent fasting, I experimented with various methods, including the 5:2 diet and alternate-day fasting. While these approaches offered some benefits, I ultimately found that the 16/8 method was the most sustainable and enjoyable for me. Trust your intuition and listen to your body's signals as you explore different fasting methods.

Seeking Support and Guidance

Embarking on an intermittent fasting journey can feel daunting, especially if you're navigating it alone. Seek support from friends, family members, or online communities who share your interest in intermittent fasting. Additionally, consider consulting with a registered dietitian, fasting coach, or healthcare provider for personalized guidance and support. Personally, I found tremendous support and encouragement from online forums and social media groups dedicated to intermittent fasting. Sharing experiences, tips, and challenges with like-minded individuals helped me stay motivated and committed to my fasting goals.

Setting Realistic Goals

Realistic goals provide direction, motivation, and a roadmap for progress. They help you stay focused, track your achievements, and celebrate your successes along the way. By setting achievable goals, you set yourself up for sustainable long-term success and avoid the pitfalls of unrealistic expectations.

Practical Tips for Setting Realistic Goals

Now, let's explore some practical tips to help you set realistic goals and maximize your intermittent fasting journey:

1. Reflect on Your Why: Start by reflecting on your reasons for embarking on an intermittent fasting journey. What are your health goals? What motivates you to make a change? Understanding your underlying motivations will help you set goals that are meaningful and aligned with your values.

- Tip: Before starting intermittent fasting, I reflected on my desire to improve my overall health, boost my energy levels, and achieve a healthy weight. Keeping these motivations in mind helped me set realistic goals that resonated with my aspirations.

2. Be Specific and Measurable: Set clear and specific goals that are easy to track and measure. Instead of setting vague goals like "lose weight," specify how much weight you

want to lose and by when. This allows you to track your progress and adjust your approach as needed.

- Tip: Instead of saying, "I want to lose weight," I set a specific goal to lose 10 pounds within the next three months. This gave me a clear target to work towards and allowed me to monitor my progress along the way.

3. Break It Down: Break down your larger goals into smaller, manageable milestones. This makes your goals feel more achievable and allows you to celebrate your progress along the way. Each milestone serves as a stepping stone towards your ultimate goal.

- Tip: If your goal is to lose 20 pounds, break it down into smaller increments, such as losing 2-3 pounds per week. Celebrate each pound lost as a milestone towards your larger goal, keeping you motivated and encouraged.

4. Set Realistic Timeframes: Be realistic about the time it will take to achieve your goals. Avoid setting arbitrary deadlines or expecting overnight transformations. Sustainable progress takes time, so be patient and trust the process.

- Tip: Instead of expecting to lose 20 pounds in a month, set a more realistic timeframe of six months to achieve your weight loss goal. This allows you focus on making gradual, sustainable changes to your lifestyle.

5. Focus on Non-Scale Victories: Shift your focus from the number on the scale to other markers of progress, such as improved energy levels, better sleep, or increased strength and endurance. Non-scale victories are equally important indicators of success and can provide motivation when the scale isn't moving.

- Tip: In addition to tracking my weight loss progress, I also paid attention to other improvements in my health, such as increased energy levels, better sleep quality, and improved mood. Celebrating these non-scale victories kept me motivated and focused on the bigger picture.

6. Be Flexible and Adaptive: Be open to adjusting your goals as needed based on your progress and evolving priorities. Listen to your body's signals, adapt your approach as necessary, and don't be afraid to seek support if you encounter challenges along the way.If you find that a particular goal or approach isn't working for you, don't hesitate to reassess and make adjustments.

7. Celebrate Your Achievements: Celebrate your successes, no matter how small, and acknowledge the progress you've made towards your goals. Celebrating achievements boosts morale, reinforces positive behaviors,

and keeps you motivated to continue on your journey.

- Tip: Whenever I reached a milestone or achieved a goal, I made sure to celebrate my accomplishments. Whether it was treating myself to a healthy meal, buying a new workout outfit, or simply acknowledging my progress on or off social media, celebrating achievements helped me stay motivated and inspired to keep going.

CHAPTER 3
CREATING YOUR INTERMITTENT FASTING PLAN

Designing Your Eating Schedule

Designing an eating schedule is a critical component of creating an effective intermittent fasting plan. Your eating schedule dictates when you consume your meals and snacks within the context of intermittent fasting, helping you structure your day and optimize the benefits of fasting.

Before designing your eating schedule, take some time to reflect on your lifestyle, preferences, and health goals. Consider factors such as your work schedule, family commitments, exercise routine, and any dietary restrictions or preferences you may have. Clarifying your objectives and understanding your lifestyle constraints will help you tailor your eating schedule to suit your individual needs and priorities.

Practical Tips for Designing Your Eating Schedule

1. Identify Your Eating Window: Determine the length of your eating window, which is the time frame during which you'll consume your meals and snacks. Consider factors such as your daily schedule, hunger levels, and energy

needs when selecting your eating window duration. Aim for a window that aligns with your natural eating patterns and allows you to feel satisfied and energized throughout the day.

- Tip: If you have a hectic schedule, opt for a condensed eating window, such as 6-8 hours, to maximize the benefits of intermittent fasting while still accommodating your lifestyle. Experiment with different window lengths to find what works best for you.

2. Plan Your Meals and Snacks: Once you've established your eating window, plan your meals and snacks accordingly. Focus on incorporating nutrient-dense foods that provide essential vitamins, minerals, and macronutrients to support your health and well-being. Aim for a balance of protein, healthy fats, fiber, and carbohydrates to keep you feeling satisfied and fueled throughout the day.

- Tip: Simplify meal planning by preparing batch-friendly recipes that can be made in advance and stored for quick and easy meals throughout the week. Invest in time-saving kitchen gadgets, such as a slow cooker or Instant Pot, to streamline meal preparation and minimize time spent in the kitchen.

3. Consider Meal Timing: Pay attention to the timing of your meals and snacks within your

eating window to optimize energy levels, digestion, and satiety. Aim to consume larger, more substantial meals earlier in the day when your body's metabolism is more active and taper off with lighter meals or snacks as the day progresses.

- Tip: Schedule your largest meal of the day during midday or early afternoon to take advantage of your body's natural circadian rhythms and optimize digestion and nutrient absorption. Keep evening meals lighter and avoid heavy or rich foods close to bedtime to promote better sleep quality.

4. Stay Hydrated: Don't forget to prioritize hydration throughout the day, especially during fasting periods. Aim to drink plenty of water, herbal tea, or other non-caloric beverages to support hydration, promote detoxification, and stave off hunger between meals.

- Tip: Keep a reusable water bottle with you throughout the day to remind yourself to stay hydrated and track your water intake. Infuse your water with slices of lemon, cucumber, or fresh herbs for added flavor and refreshment.

5. Listen when your body speaks: Above all, listen to your body's cues and adjust your eating schedule as needed based on hunger, energy levels, and overall well-being. Be flexible and willing to experiment with

different approaches until you find what works best for you and supports your health goals.

- Tip: Pay attention to how your body responds to intermittent fasting and adjust your eating schedule accordingly. If you find that certain eating windows or meal timings leave you feeling overly hungry or fatigued, consider modifying your approach to better suit your needs and lifestyle.

Meal Planning and Preparation

Meal planning and preparation are essential components of creating a successful intermittent fasting plan. By carefully selecting and preparing your meals in advance, you can ensure that you have nutritious options readily available during your eating window, streamline your mealtime routine, and support your health goals.Meal planning and preparation play a crucial role in intermittent fasting by helping you make informed food choices, manage portion sizes, and stay on track with your health goals. By taking the time to plan and prepare your meals ahead of time, you can reduce the temptation to make impulsive food choices, save time and money, and minimize stress associated with mealtime decisions. Additionally, meal planning and preparation allow you to incorporate a variety of nutrient-dense foods into your diet, ensuring that you meet your nutritional needs and support overall health and well-being.

Practical Tips for Meal Planning and Preparation

- Set Aside Time for Planning: Schedule dedicated time each week to plan your meals and snacks. Create a meal plan for the week, outlining breakfast, lunch, dinner, and any snacks or desserts you'd like to includeConsider factors such as your eating window, dietary preferences, and nutritional needs when selecting recipes and creating your meal plan. Use tools such as meal planning apps or printable templates to streamline the process.

- Choose Nutrient-Dense Foods: Focus on incorporating nutrient-dense foods into your meals and snacks to support your health and energy levels. Include a variety of fruits, vegetables, whole grains, lean proteins, and healthy fats to ensure you're meeting your nutritional needs. Aim for a balance of macronutrients (carbohydrates, proteins, and fats) and micronutrients (vitamins and minerals) in each meal.
- Shop with a List: Before heading to the grocery store, make a list of all the ingredients you'll need for your meals and snacks. Stick to your list to avoid impulse purchases and ensure that you have everything you need to execute your meal plan. Consider shopping at farmers' markets or local produce stands for fresh, seasonal ingredients.
- Batch-Cook and Prep Ingredients: Spend some time batch-cooking or prepping ingredients in advance to save time during the week. Prepare sufficient quantities of veggies, grains, and meats so they may be used for several meals over the week. Chop fruits and vegetables, portion out snacks, and

pre-measure ingredients to make meal assembly quick and easy.

- Use Time-Saving Kitchen Tools: Take advantage of time-saving kitchen tools and appliances to streamline meal preparation. Invest in a slow cooker, Instant Pot, or air fryer to cook meals quickly and efficiently. Use kitchen gadgets like vegetable slicers, food processors, and immersion blenders to simplify meal prep tasks.

- Prep Portable Snacks: Prepare portable snacks and meals that you can take with you on the go. Pack individual portions of nuts, seeds, dried fruit, or trail mix for quick and convenient snacks. Make homemade energy bars, protein balls, or veggie sticks with hummus for satisfying on-the-go options.

- Focus on Variety and Flavor: Keep your meals interesting and flavorful by incorporating a variety of ingredients, spices, and seasonings. Experiment with different cuisines, cooking methods, and flavor combinations to keep your taste buds excited and engaged. Consider trying new recipes or incorporating seasonal produce for added variety.

- Consider Convenience: Choose recipes and meal options that are convenient and easy to prepare, especially on busy days. Look for quick and simple recipes that require minimal ingredients and cooking time, such as sheet pan meals, one-pot dishes, or make-ahead salads. Stock your pantry with staple ingredients that can be used to whip up quick and nutritious meals on the fly.

- Listen to body signals: Pay attention to how your body responds to different foods and eating patterns, and adjust your meal plan accordingly. Notice how certain foods make you feel and prioritize those that leave you feeling satisfied, energized, and nourished. Be flexible and willing to adapt your meal plan based on your changing needs and preferences.

Choosing The Best Diet For Intermittent Fasting

In addition to meal planning and preparation, choosing the best diet to complement your intermittent fasting approach is crucial for achieving your health goals. While there is no one-size-fits-all diet that works for everyone, there are some general principles to consider when selecting a diet that aligns with intermittent fasting:

- Focus on Whole, Unprocessed Foods: Choose whole, unprocessed foods as the foundation of your diet, including fruits, vegetables, whole grains, lean proteins, and healthy fats. These foods are rich in essential nutrients, fiber, and antioxidants, and can help support overall health and well-being.
- Prioritize Protein: Incorporate protein-rich foods into your meals and snacks to support muscle repair, satiety, and metabolism. Aim for a balance of plant-based and animal-based protein sources, such as beans, lentils, tofu, tempeh, poultry, fish, eggs, and dairy products.
- Include Healthy Fats: Incorporate foods like avocados, nuts, seeds, olive oil, and fatty fish into your diet as sources of healthy fats. Healthy fats provide essential fatty acids, vitamins, and minerals, and help promote satiety and stabilize blood sugar levels.

- Limit Added Sugars and Processed Foods: Minimize your intake of added sugars, refined carbohydrates, and processed foods, which can contribute to inflammation, insulin resistance, and weight gain. Opt for whole, nutrient-dense foods whenever possible and read labels carefully to avoid hidden sources of added sugars and unhealthy additives.
- Stay Hydrated: Drink plenty of water throughout the day to stay hydrated and support overall health and well-being. Water is essential for digestion, metabolism, and cellular function, and can help prevent dehydration, which can negatively impact energy levels and cognitive function.

Best Diets for Intermittent Fasting

While there is no one-size-fits-all approach, several dietary patterns are commonly used in conjunction with intermittent fasting. Here are some popular options:

- Mediterranean Diet: The focus of the Mediterranean diet is on whole foods that have undergone minimal processing, including fruits, vegetables, whole grains, legumes, nuts, seeds, and olive oil. It also contains dairy, red wine, poultry, and fish in moderation. This diet is rich in nutrients, antioxidants, and healthy fats, making it a popular choice for supporting overall health and well-being.

- Low-Carb or Keto Diet: Low-carb and keto diets restrict carbohydrate intake while emphasizing high-fat and moderate protein foods. These diets promote ketosis, a metabolic state in which the body burns fat for fuel. They are often used in conjunction with intermittent fasting to enhance fat burning and support weight loss.
- Plant-Based Diet: A plant-based diet focuses on whole, plant foods such as fruits, vegetables, legumes, nuts, seeds, and whole grains. It excludes or minimizes animal products, making it rich in fiber, vitamins, minerals, and antioxidants. Plant-based diets are associated with numerous health benefits, including improved heart health, weight management, and longevity.
- Paleo Diet: The Paleo diet mimics the eating patterns of our hunter-gatherer ancestors, emphasizing whole, unprocessed foods such as meat, fish, eggs, fruits, vegetables, nuts, and seeds. It excludes grains, legumes, dairy, and processed foods, making it rich in protein, healthy fats, and micronutrients.

When choosing the best diet for you, consider your individual preferences, dietary restrictions, and health goals.

Tracking Progress and Adjusting as Needed

Tracking progress provides valuable insights into the effectiveness of your intermittent fasting plan and helps you stay accountable to your goals. By monitoring key metrics such as weight, body measurements, energy levels, and dietary habits, you can identify patterns, track changes over time, and make informed decisions about your health and wellness journey. Additionally, tracking progress allows you to celebrate successes, stay motivated, and course-correct if necessary to ensure continued progress towards your goals.

There are several methods you can use to track your progress with intermittent fasting. They include:

1. Keep a Food Journal: Record what you eat and drink each day, along with the timing of your meals and fasting periods. Note any cravings, hunger levels, and mood changes to identify patterns and trends over time. Keeping a food journal can help you become more mindful of your eating habits and make adjustments as needed to support your goals.

2. Use a Weight Scale: Regularly weigh yourself using a reliable scale and track your weight over time. While fluctuations are normal, monitoring your weight can help you assess

the effectiveness of your intermittent fasting plan and make adjustments if your progress stalls or plateaus. Remember to weigh yourself under consistent conditions, such as first thing in the morning before eating or drinking.

3. Measure Body Composition: In addition to weight, consider tracking other measures of body composition, such as body measurements, body fat percentage, and muscle mass. Use a tape measure to record measurements of key areas, such as waist, hips, thighs, and arms, and track changes over time. This can provide a more comprehensive picture of your progress beyond just weight loss.

4. Monitor Energy Levels and Well-Being: Pay attention to how you feel physically, mentally, and emotionally throughout the day. Notice changes in energy levels, mood, and cognitive function, and assess how these factors are impacted by your intermittent fasting plan. Keeping a journal or diary can help you track these subjective measures and identify patterns or triggers that may affect your well-being.

5. Use Technology: Take advantage of technology to simplify tracking and analysis. There are numerous apps and tools available that can help you track food intake, monitor

physical activity, record weight and measurements, and even analyze sleep patterns and stress levels. Find a tool that aligns with your preferences and goals and use it consistently to track your progress.

Strategies for Adjusting Your Intermittent Fasting Plan

When I first started intermittent fasting, I was excited about the potential health benefits but unsure of how to track my progress effectively. I began by keeping a food journal, recording my meals, fasting periods, and any notable observations about my eating habits and hunger levels. I also weighed myself regularly and measured my body composition using a tape measure.As I continued with intermittent fasting, I noticed gradual changes in my weight and body measurements, as well as improvements in my energy levels and overall well-being. However, I also encountered challenges along the way, such as cravings, mood swings, and fluctuations in energy.To address these challenges, I experimented with different eating windows, meal timings, and food choices to see how they impacted my progress and well-being. I adjusted my meal plan based on my observations and feedback from my body, focusing on nutrient-dense foods, balanced meals, and adequate hydration.Over time, I found a rhythm that worked well for me, incorporating regular fasting periods, nourishing meals, and mindful eating practices into my daily routine. By tracking my progress and adjusting my approach as needed, I was able to achieve my health goals, maintain a healthy weight, and experience the many benefits of intermittent fasting.

Based on my personal experience and research, here are some strategies for adjusting your intermittent fasting plan as needed:

1. Be Flexible: Intermittent fasting is not one-size-fits-all, and what works for one person may not work for another. Be open to experimentation and willing to adapt your approach based on your individual needs and preferences.

2. Listen to Your Body: Pay attention to how your body responds to different eating patterns, meal timings, and food choices. Notice any changes in hunger, energy levels, mood, and well-being, and adjust your plan accordingly.

3. Gradual Changes: Implement changes to your intermittent fasting plan gradually, rather than making drastic adjustments all at once. This allows your body to adapt slowly and minimizes the risk of negative side effects or disruptions to your routine.

4. Seek Support: Don't hesitate to seek support from healthcare professionals, registered dietitians, or certified nutritionists if you're struggling with your intermittent fasting plan or need personalized guidance. They can provide expert advice and tailored recommendations to help you achieve your health goals.

5. Be Consistent: When it comes to intermittent fasting, consistency is essential. Stick to your eating schedule and fasting periods as much as possible, even on weekends or holidays. This helps maintain metabolic stability and supports long-term success with intermittent fasting.

CHAPTER 4
MAKING INTERMITTEN T
FASTING EASY AND SUSTAINABLE

Strategies for managing hunger and cravings during fasting periods

Hunger and cravings are common experiences during fasting periods, but they are distinct sensations that arise from different physiological and psychological mechanisms.

Hunger is the body's natural response to the absence of food, signaling a need for nourishment. It is often accompanied by physical symptoms such as stomach growling, low energy levels, and a gnawing sensation in the stomach. Hunger typically subsides after eating and is regulated by hormones such as ghrelin, which stimulates appetite.

Cravings, on the other hand, are intense desires for specific foods or flavors, often unrelated to actual hunger. Cravings can be triggered by various factors, including emotions, stress, environmental cues, and habitual patterns of eating. They are influenced by neurotransmitters such as dopamine, which plays a role in reward-seeking behavior.

While hunger is a natural and necessary physiological response to fasting, cravings can be more challenging to manage as they are often driven by psychological and emotional factors. By understanding the differences between hunger and cravings, you can develop strategies to address each effectively and navigate fasting periods with greater ease.

Strategies for Managing Hunger During Fasting Periods

Here are some practical strategies to help you manage hunger during fasting periods:

1. Stay Hydrated: Drinking water or other non-caloric beverages can help reduce feelings of hunger and keep you hydrated during fasting periods. Aim to drink at least 8-10 glasses of water per day, and consider incorporating herbal tea, black coffee, or sparkling water to add variety to your hydration routine.
2. Consume Fiber-Rich Foods: Foods high in fiber, such as fruits, vegetables, whole grains, and legumes, can help promote feelings of fullness and satiety. Include plenty of fiber-rich foods in your meals and snacks during eating windows to help you feel satisfied for longer periods.

3. Prioritize Protein: Protein is known for its ability to promote satiety and support muscle maintenance and repair. Include lean sources of protein, such as poultry, fish, eggs, tofu, and legumes, in your meals to help you feel full and satisfied during fasting periods.

4. Incorporate Healthy Fats: Healthy fats, such as those found in avocados, nuts, seeds, olive oil, and fatty fish, can help slow digestion and promote feelings of fullness. Include a serving of healthy fats in your meals to help you stay satisfied throughout the day.

5. Practice Mindful Eating: Pay attention to your hunger and fullness cues, and eat mindfully during eating windows. Chew your food slowly, savoring each bite, and stop eating when you feel satisfied rather than overly full. Avoid distractions, such as watching TV or scrolling on your phone, while eating to help you tune into your body's signals.

Strategies for Managing Cravings During Fasting Periods

1. Identify Triggers: Pay attention to what triggers your cravings, whether it's stress, boredom, emotions, or environmental cues. By identifying your triggers, you can develop strategies to address them and reduce the likelihood of experiencing cravings.

2. Distract Yourself: When cravings strike, distract yourself with activities that engage your mind and body. Go for a walk, practice deep breathing exercises, or engage in a hobby or activity that you enjoy to take your mind off food cravings.

3. Practice Delayed Gratification: Instead of giving in to cravings immediately, practice delaying gratification by waiting a set amount of time before indulging. During this time, distract yourself with other activities or focus on your goals and reasons for fasting to help you resist the temptation to give in to cravings.

4. Choose Healthy Alternatives: If you're craving a specific food, try to find a healthier alternative that satisfies your craving without derailing your fasting plan. For example, if you're craving something sweet, reach for a piece of fruit or a small serving of dark chocolate instead of sugary snacks or desserts.

5. Plan Ahead: Anticipate cravings and plan ahead by having healthy snacks and meals prepared and readily available during fasting periods. Choose nutrient-dense foods that will help keep you satisfied and energized until your next meal.

What to Eat During Your Eating Windows: Nutrient-dense Meal Planning

Nutrient-dense meal planning involves choosing foods that are rich in essential nutrients, including vitamins, minerals, fiber, and antioxidants, while limiting processed foods, added sugars, and unhealthy fats. By prioritizing nutrient-dense foods, you can fuel your body with the nutrients it needs to function optimally and support your health goals.

The Benefits of Nutrient-Dense Meal Planning

- Promotes Overall Health: Nutrient-dense foods provide the essential vitamins, minerals, and antioxidants needed for optimal health. A diet rich in nutrient-dense foods has been linked to reduced risk of chronic diseases such as heart disease, diabetes, and certain cancers.

- Supports Weight Management: Nutrient-dense foods are typically lower in calories and higher in fiber, which can help you feel fuller for longer and reduce overall calorie intake. Incorporating nutrient-dense foods into your meals can support weight management and help you achieve your desired body composition.

- Enhances Energy Levels: Nutrient-dense foods provide a steady source of energy and help stabilize blood sugar levels throughout the day. By choosing nutrient-dense options, you can avoid energy crashes and maintain consistent energy levels to support daily activities and exercise.
- Improves Digestive Health: Foods rich in fiber, such as fruits, vegetables, whole grains, and legumes, support digestive health by promoting regularity and preventing constipation. Including fiber-rich foods in your meals can support a healthy gut microbiome and reduce the risk of digestive disorders.

Practical Tips for Nutrient-Dense Meal Planning

- Prioritize Whole Foods: Focus on including a variety of whole, minimally processed foods in your meals, such as fruits, vegetables, whole grains, lean proteins, and healthy fats. These foods are naturally rich in nutrients and provide essential vitamins, minerals, and antioxidants to support overall health.
- Include a Variety of Colors: Aim to incorporate a rainbow of colors into your meals by choosing fruits and vegetables of different hues. Each color represents different nutrients and antioxidants, so including a

variety ensures you're getting a broad spectrum of nutrients to support your health.

- Balance Macronutrients: Aim to include a balance of carbohydrates, proteins, and fats in each meal to provide sustained energy and satiety. Incorporate complex carbohydrates, such as whole grains and starchy vegetables, lean proteins, such as poultry, fish, tofu, and legumes, and healthy fats, such as avocados, nuts, seeds, and olive oil.

- Choose Quality Protein Sources: Opt for lean sources of protein, such as poultry, fish, eggs, tofu, and legumes, to support muscle maintenance and repair. Include a serving of protein in each meal to help you feel full and satisfied and support muscle recovery after exercise.

- Include Healthy Fats: Incorporate healthy fats, such as avocados, nuts, seeds, olive oil, and fatty fish, into your meals to support heart health and promote satiety. Choose unsaturated fats over saturated and trans fats and limit sources of unhealthy fats, such as processed and fried foods.

- Plan Ahead: To guarantee that you have nutrient-dense options on hand during your eating window, make the time to plan your meals and snacks in advance. Stock your kitchen with healthy staples, such as fresh produce, whole grains, lean proteins, and healthy fats, and prepare meals and snacks in batches to save time during busy days.

Sample Nutrient-Dense Meal Ideas

Here are some examples of nutrient-dense meals to inspire your meal planning:

Breakfast:

Overnight oats topped with fresh berries, sliced almonds, and a drizzle of honey

Greek yogurt with granola, sliced banana, and a sprinkle of chia seeds

Lunch:

Quinoa salad with mixed greens, cherry tomatoes, cucumber, avocado, chickpeas, and grilled chicken

Lentil soup with whole grain bread and a side salad with balsamic vinaigrette

Dinner:

Baked salmon with roasted sweet potatoes and steamed broccoli

Stir-fried tofu with mixed vegetables served over brown rice

Snacks:

Sliced apple with almond butter

Carrot sticks with hummus

Trail mix made with nuts, seeds, and dried fruit

Breakfast:

Scrambled eggs with spinach, bell peppers, onions, and feta cheese

Whole grain toast with mashed avocado and sliced tomato

Lunch:

Quinoa and black bean salad with corn, red onion, cilantro, and lime vinaigrette

Grilled veggie wrap with mixed greens and hummus

Dinner:

Quinoa pilaf, grilled chicken breast, and steamed asparagus

Spaghetti squash with marinara sauce and turkey meatballs

Snacks:

Greek yogurt topped with granola and chopped peaches

Cottage cheese with pineapple chunks

Breakfast:

Whole grain waffles topped with Greek yogurt, mixed berries, and a drizzle of maple syrup

Breakfast burrito with scrambled eggs, black beans, avocado, and salsa wrapped in a whole grain tortilla

Lunch:

Mixed green salad with grilled shrimp, mango, avocado, and lime-cilantro dressing

Veggie-packed quinoa bowl with roasted vegetables, edamame, avocado, and tahini dressing

Staying hydrated: Importance of water and other beverages during fasting

Water is the essence of life, playing a pivotal role in maintaining bodily functions and processes. During fasting, when the body relies on stored energy reserves, proper hydration becomes even more vital. Fasting can lead to increased water loss through various channels, including urine, sweat, and respiration. Therefore, staying hydrated is essential to support the body's needs and prevent dehydration, which can lead to various health complications.

The Role of Hydration

Maintaining hydration levels during intermittent fasting is crucial for several reasons:

- Sustained Energy Levels: Proper hydration helps combat fatigue and sluggishness, allowing you to stay energized and focused throughout the day, even during fasting periods.
- Supporting Hormonal Balance: Hydration plays a role in hormone regulation, which is especially important for women over forty who may experience hormonal changes associated with perimenopause or menopause. Adequate hydration can help

alleviate symptoms such as hot flashes and mood swings.

- Optimizing Cognitive Function: Dehydration can impair cognitive function, affecting memory, concentration, and overall mental clarity. By staying hydrated, busy women can maintain optimal cognitive function and productivity.
- Promoting Digestive Health: Hydration supports proper digestion and bowel function, helping prevent constipation and promoting regularity, which is essential for overall digestive health, particularly as women age.
- Maintaining Fluid Balance: Adequate hydration helps maintain fluid balance in the body, ensuring that essential functions, such as blood circulation and nutrient transport, can occur efficiently.
- Supporting Detoxification: Water plays a crucial role in the detoxification process, helping flush toxins and waste products from the body through urine and sweat. Staying hydrated during fasting can support this process and promote overall detoxification.
- Preventing Fatigue and Headaches: Dehydration can lead to symptoms such as fatigue, headaches, and dizziness, which can interfere with your ability to function optimally during fasting periods. By staying hydrated, you can minimize these symptoms

and maintain energy levels throughout the day.

- Supporting Weight Loss: Drinking water can help promote feelings of fullness and satiety, reducing the likelihood of overeating during eating windows and supporting weight loss goals.

Practical Tips for Staying Hydrated During Fasting

Here are some practical tips for staying hydrated during fasting periods:

1. Set Hydration Goals: Aim to drink a certain amount of water each day, such as 8-10 glasses, to ensure you're meeting your hydration needs. Keep track of your water intake using a water tracking app or simply by carrying a reusable water bottle and refilling it throughout the day.

2. Hydrate Upon Waking: Start your day by drinking a glass of water as soon as you wake up. This helps kickstart your metabolism, rehydrate your body after sleep, and sets a positive tone for the rest of the day.

3. Incorporate Electrolytes: Electrolytes play a crucial role in hydration and are especially important during fasting periods. Consider adding electrolyte-rich foods and beverages to your diet, such as coconut water, leafy greens,

and electrolyte-enhanced drinks, to replenish lost electrolytes and maintain proper hydration levels.

4. Sip Herbal Teas: Herbal teas are hydrating and can provide additional health benefits. Choose caffeine-free options such as chamomile, peppermint, or ginger tea, which can help promote relaxation, aid digestion, and alleviate stress.

5. Snack on Hydrating Foods: Incorporate hydrating foods into your meals and snacks, such as fruits and vegetables with high water content, including cucumbers, watermelon, strawberries, and celery. These foods not only contribute to your overall hydration but also provide essential nutrients and antioxidants.

6. Avoid Excessive Caffeine and Alcohol: Limit your intake of caffeinated beverages and alcoholic drinks, as they can have a diuretic effect and contribute to dehydration. Opt for water or herbal teas as your primary sources of hydration, especially during fasting periods.

7. Pay attention to your body: Drink water when you feel thirsty and pay attention to your body's thirst signals. Additionally, be mindful of other signs of dehydration, such as dry mouth, dark urine, fatigue, and headaches, and respond promptly by increasing your fluid intake.

8. Plan Ahead: Prepare hydrating beverages and snacks in advance to have them readily available during fasting periods. Keep a variety of hydrating options on hand, such as infused water, herbal teas, and electrolyte drinks, to ensure you have choices that appeal to you throughout the day.

Healthy Beverages for Women Over 40

In addition to water, there are several healthy beverages that are especially beneficial for women over 40 during fasting periods:

- Green Tea: Green tea is rich in antioxidants and has been associated with numerous health benefits, including improved heart health, weight management, and reduced inflammation. It also contains a small amount of caffeine, which can help boost energy levels during fasting periods.
- Bone Broth: Bone broth is a nutritious and hydrating beverage that is rich in protein, collagen, and essential nutrients such as calcium, magnesium, and phosphorus. It can help support gut health, joint health, and overall immunity during fasting periods.
- Coconut Water: Coconut water is a natural source of electrolytes, including potassium, sodium, and magnesium, making it an excellent choice for hydration during fasting.

It's low in calories and sugar, making it suitable for those watching their calorie intake.

- Vegetable Juice: Freshly squeezed vegetable juices are a nutrient-dense and hydrating option during fasting periods. They provide essential vitamins, minerals, and antioxidants, while also keeping you hydrated and satisfied.
- Herbal Infusions: Herbal infusions such as hibiscus, rooibos, and nettle tea are caffeine-free and hydrating options that offer various health benefits. They can help support digestion, reduce inflammation, and promote relaxation during fasting periods.

Staying hydrated is essential for maintaining health and well-being, especially during intermittent fasting. By prioritizing hydration and incorporating practical strategies and healthy beverages into your fasting plan, you can support your body's needs, prevent dehydration, and maximize the benefits of intermittent fasting. Remember to drink plenty of water, include electrolyte-rich foods and beverages, and listen to your body's thirst signals to stay properly hydrated throughout the day.

Exercise and Intermittent Fasting

Exercise and intermittent fasting are two powerful tools for improving health and well-being. When combined, they can enhance each other's benefits. Before delving into how they work together, let me share my journey with incorporating exercise into my fasting routine.

Initially, like many, I found the idea of exercising while fasting daunting. I worried about feeling weak or lightheaded during workouts, unsure if I could perform at my best without fueling up beforehand. But after some research and consulting with a healthcare professional, I decided to give it a shot.Starting small was key for me. In my early forties and not particularly keen on working out, I began with early morning walks, gradually adding morning and evening sessions. As I grew more comfortable, I progressed to jogging in the mornings and walking in the evenings.

During my research, I stumbled upon high-intensity interval training (HIIT). Although intrigued, I was unsure how to approach it. About a year into intermittent fasting, feeling energetic and ready for a change, I ventured into HIIT through YouTube channels, fitting it into my evening routine. The flexibility of online videos allowed me to work at my own pace, gradually mastering the exercises. I experimented with various trainers before settling on two who suited me best. Encouraged by a friend, I delved into weight training. Navigating this new territory cautiously, I joined a gym and sought the guidance of a personal trainer to ensure safety and effectiveness.

I share my experience to reassure you that starting small is okay. Whether it's a walk or a skip, find something that keeps you active. Despite busy schedules, dedicating just thirty minutes to a daily walk or jog yields significant results over time. Know that this is a marathon, not a sprint. Pace yourselves and embrace the process.

Benefits of Exercise and Intermittent fasting

Exercise and intermittent fasting both have unique effects on the body, but when combined, they can produce synergistic benefits. Let's take a closer look at how exercise and intermittent fasting influence various aspects of health:

- Weight Management: Both exercise and intermittent fasting can help support weight loss and weight management efforts. Exercise increases energy expenditure and promotes fat loss, while intermittent fasting enhances fat burning and metabolic efficiency.
- Metabolic Health: Exercise has been shown to improve insulin sensitivity, reduce

inflammation, and promote metabolic health. Intermittent fasting also has metabolic benefits, such as lowering insulin levels, improving blood sugar control, and supporting cellular repair processes.

- Energy Levels: Contrary to common belief, exercising while fasting can actually increase energy levels and enhance workout performance for some individuals. Fasting promotes the use of stored fat for fuel, leading to sustained energy levels and improved endurance during exercise.

- Muscle Preservation: Concerns about muscle loss during fasting are often overstated, especially when combined with resistance training. In fact, intermittent fasting may help preserve lean muscle mass by promoting the release of growth hormone and enhancing muscle protein synthesis.

- Mental Clarity: Many people report improved mental clarity and focus when exercising while fasting. This may be due to increased adrenaline and cortisol levels, which can sharpen cognitive function and enhance alertness during workouts.

Incorporating Exercise into Your Fasting Routine

Now that we understand the potential benefits of exercising while fasting, let's discuss how to incorporate exercise into your fasting routine effectively:

1. Choose the Right Type of Exercise: Focus on low to moderate-intensity activities such as walking, jogging, cycling, swimming, or yoga during fasting periods. Save high-intensity or strenuous workouts for your eating windows when you have adequate fuel and energy.

2. Listen to Your Body: Pay attention to how you feel during workouts and adjust your intensity level accordingly. If you feel weak, lightheaded, or dizzy, take a break and refuel with water or a small snack if necessary.

3. Stay Hydrated: Hydration is essential when exercising while fasting. Drink plenty of water before, during, and after workouts to stay hydrated and support optimal performance.

4. Time Your Workouts Wisely: Schedule your workouts strategically to align with your fasting and eating windows. Some people prefer to exercise in the morning before breaking their fast, while others find it more comfortable to exercise later in the day after consuming their first meal.

5. Fuel Up Appropriately: If you plan to engage in prolonged or intense exercise sessions, consider consuming a small snack or meal containing carbohydrates and protein before your workout to provide your body with sufficient energy and nutrients.

6. Focus on Recovery: Pay attention to post-workout recovery by consuming a balanced meal containing protein, carbohydrates, and healthy fats to replenish glycogen stores and support muscle repair and growth.

Understanding Weight Training and HIT Workouts

Using resistance to increase muscular strength and endurance is known as weight training, commonly referred to as resistance training or strength training. This type of exercise typically involves lifting weights or using resistance bands to perform exercises targeting specific muscle groups.

High-intensity interval training (HIT) workouts involve alternating between short bursts of intense exercise and periods of rest or lower-intensity activity. These workouts are designed to maximize calorie burn, improve cardiovascular fitness, and boost metabolism in a shorter amount of time compared to steady-state cardio exercises.

Both weight training and HIT workouts offer numerous benefits when incorporated into an intermittent fasting routine:

- Preservation of Lean Muscle Mass: Weight training helps preserve lean muscle mass while promoting fat loss during fasting periods. Maintaining muscle mass is essential for overall health, metabolism, and physical function, especially as we age.
- Increased Calorie Burn: Both weight training and HIT workouts can increase calorie expenditure both during and after exercise, leading to greater fat loss and improved body composition over time.
- Metabolic Adaptation: Intense workouts like HIT can enhance metabolic adaptation, leading to improved insulin sensitivity, enhanced fat oxidation, and better overall metabolic health.
- Improved Strength and Endurance: Weight training improves muscular strength and endurance, making everyday tasks easier and reducing the risk of injury. HIT workouts can also improve cardiovascular fitness and endurance, leading to better overall physical performance.
- Enhanced Mood and Mental Health: Exercise releases endorphins, which can improve mood, reduce stress, and enhance mental

well-being, all of which are important during fasting periods.

Practical Tips for Incorporating Weight Training and HIT Workouts While Fasting

Here are some practical tips for incorporating weight training and HIT workouts into your fasting routine:

- Choose the Right Time: Schedule your workouts during your eating window or shortly before breaking your fast to ensure you have enough energy and nutrients to fuel your workout and support recovery afterward.
- Stay Hydrated: Hydration is crucial when exercising while fasting. Stay hydrated and promote optimal performance by drinking lots of water prior to, during, and after exercises.
- Start Slowly: If you're new to weight training or HIT workouts, start with lighter weights and shorter intervals, gradually increasing intensity and duration as you build strength and endurance.
- Focus on Compound Movements: Incorporate compound exercises that target multiple muscle groups simultaneously, such as squats, deadlifts, bench presses, and rows. These exercises are efficient and effective for building strength and muscle mass.

- Include Rest Days: Allow for adequate rest and recovery between workouts to prevent overtraining and reduce the risk of injury. Pay attention to your body's needs and modify the frequency and intensity of your workouts accordingly.
- Fuel Up After Workouts: Consume a balanced meal containing protein, carbohydrates, and healthy fats after your workout to replenish glycogen stores, support muscle repair and growth, and enhance recovery.
- Be Consistent: Consistency is key when it comes to seeing results from weight training and HIT workouts. Aim to incorporate these types of exercise into your fasting routine regularly, ideally at least 2-3 times per week.
- Listen to Your Body: : While fasting, observe how your body reacts to exercise. If you feel weak, dizzy, or excessively fatigued, take a break and refuel with a small snack.

By following these practical tips and staying consistent with your exercise regimen, you can build strength, improve endurance, and optimize your health and well-being while fasting.

CHAPTER 5

OVERCOMING COMMON CHALLENGES

Dealing with Social Situations and Social Pressure

Social situations, such as family gatherings, parties, dinners with friends, and workplace events, often revolve around food. These occasions can present challenges for individuals following an intermittent fasting protocol, as they may feel pressured to eat outside of their designated eating windows or break their fast prematurely.

Social pressure can come from various sources, including well-meaning friends and family members who may not understand or support your fasting goals. Peer pressure to indulge in unhealthy foods or participate in frequent eating can make it difficult to adhere to your fasting schedule and stay on track with your dietary goals.

Practical Tips for Dealing with Social Situations and Social Pressure

1. Communicate Your Goals: Be upfront and transparent with friends and family members

about your intermittent fasting regimen and the reasons behind it. Educate them about the health benefits of fasting and how it aligns with your personal goals. By setting clear boundaries and expectations, you can enlist their support and understanding.

2. Plan Ahead: Before attending social events, plan your fasting and eating schedule accordingly. If possible, schedule your eating window to coincide with the event, allowing you to enjoy the festivities without feeling pressured to deviate from your fasting regimen. Alternatively, consider adjusting your fasting schedule on the day of the event to accommodate social eating while still adhering to your overall fasting goals.

3. Bring Your Own Food: If you're concerned about the availability of fasting-friendly options at social gatherings, consider bringing your own food or snacks that align with your dietary preferences. This ensures that you have healthy options to enjoy during the event and reduces the temptation to indulge in less nutritious foods.

4. Focus on Non-Food Activities: Shift the focus of social gatherings away from food by suggesting alternative activities such as going for a walk, playing games, or engaging in conversation. By redirecting attention away from eating, you can enjoy social interactions

without feeling pressured to consume food outside of your fasting window.

5. Practice Mindful Eating: If you do choose to eat during social events, practice mindful eating by savoring each bite, eating slowly, and paying attention to hunger and fullness cues. Avoid mindless snacking or overeating due to social pressure, and prioritize nourishing foods that align with your dietary goals.

6. Be Firm but Polite: If friends or family members pressure you to break your fast or indulge in unhealthy foods, politely but firmly assert your boundaries. You can simply say, "No thank you, I'm fasting right now," or "I appreciate the offer, but I'm choosing to stick to my eating schedule."

7. Seek Support: Surround yourself with like-minded individuals who understand and support your intermittent fasting goals. Join online communities, forums, or social media groups where you can connect with others following similar dietary approaches and share experiences, tips, and encouragement.

8. Practice Self-Compassion: Remember that intermittent fasting is a personal choice, and it's okay to deviate from your fasting schedule occasionally. Don't be too hard on yourself if you slip up or indulge in food outside of your eating window. Instead, practice

self-compassion and focus on getting back on track with your fasting goals.

9. Emotional eating is driven by psychological factors rather than physiological hunger. It often involves consuming food as a means of soothing or numbing uncomfortable emotions, seeking comfort or distraction, or rewarding oneself. Stress, worry, despair, loneliness, boredom, or even happy feelings like joy or enthusiasm can all be triggers for emotional eating.

Managing Emotional Eating

Emotional eating is the practice of using food to cope with or suppress emotions rather than to satisfy physical hunger. It often involves consuming food in response to stress, boredom, sadness, loneliness, or other emotional triggers. Many of us have experienced the urge to reach for a pint of ice cream after a stressful day at work or to indulge in a bag of chips when feeling lonely or bored.

The Impact of Emotional Eating on Intermittent Fasting

For individuals following an intermittent fasting regimen, emotional eating can disrupt their fasting schedule and undermine their efforts to achieve their health and weight loss goals. Consuming food outside of designated eating windows or succumbing to cravings triggered by emotions can lead to overeating, excessive calorie intake, and weight gain. Moreover, emotional eating can perpetuate feelings of guilt, shame, and failure, making it challenging to maintain consistency with fasting.

I have struggled with emotional eating for as long as I can remember, and incorporating intermittent fasting into my lifestyle only exacerbated the issue. During fasting periods, I found myself turning to food as a source of comfort or distraction, especially when faced with stressful situations or intense emotions. Despite my best intentions to adhere to my fasting schedule, I often succumbed to the temptation to eat outside of my designated eating window, leading to feelings of guilt and frustration.

One particularly challenging experience occurred when I received some disappointing news at work. Feeling overwhelmed and stressed, I found myself mindlessly reaching for a bag of cookies, rationalizing that I deserved a treat to help me feel better. Before I knew it, I had consumed the entire bag, breaking my fast and derailing my efforts to stick to my dietary goals. As I reflected on my behavior afterward, I realized the detrimental impact of emotional eating on my fasting goals and overall well-being. I felt disappointed in myself for succumbing to old patterns of behavior and allowing my emotions to dictate my food choices. But I also understood that it took time, self-awareness, and compassion to overcome emotional eating; it was not an easy process.

I worked hard in the days and weeks that followed to change my emotional eating patterns and create more beneficial coping skills. I sought support from friends and loved ones, confiding in them about my struggles and enlisting their encouragement and accountability. I also immersed myself in activities that brought me joy and fulfillment, such as spending time outdoors, taking long walks and dancing.

Over time, I began to notice a shift in my relationship with food and emotions. By practicing mindfulness and self-awareness, I learned to recognize the signs of emotional hunger and differentiate them from true physical hunger cues. I became more aware of my body's demands and learned techniques for handling stress and emotions without reaching for comfort food.

Today, I continue to practice intermittent fasting as part of my lifestyle, but with a newfound sense of balance and perspective. While the temptation to emotionally eat still arises from time to time, I approach it with greater mindfulness knowing that I have the tools and support system in place to navigate the challenges.

Practical Tips for Managing Emotional Eating

- Identify Triggers: Take note of the emotions, situations, or events that trigger your urge to eat. Keep a journal to monitor your eating habits and pinpoint typical emotional eating triggers. By becoming more aware of your triggers, you can develop strategies to address them effectively.
- Practice Mindfulness: Before reaching for food, pause and assess your hunger cues. Ask yourself if you're eating out of physical hunger or if you're seeking comfort or distraction from emotions. Mindful eating involves

paying attention to the sensory experience of eating and being present in the moment.

- Find Alternative Coping Mechanisms: Discover other Coping Mechanisms: To handle emotions without resorting to food, cultivate a repertoire of other coping mechanisms. Engage in activities such as deep breathing, meditation, journaling, exercise, or creative pursuits to help regulate emotions and reduce stress.

- Create a Supportive Environment: Surround yourself with supportive friends, family members, or peers who understand your intermittent fasting goals and can offer encouragement and accountability. Share your challenges and successes with others, and seek support when needed.

- Plan Ahead: Anticipate situations that may trigger emotional eating and plan ahead for how you will cope. Stock your kitchen with healthy, satisfying snacks that align with your fasting goals, and avoid keeping trigger foods in the house.

- Practice Self-Compassion: Be gentle with yourself and recognize that emotional eating is a common struggle for many individuals. Instead of berating yourself for slipping up, practice self-compassion and focus on learning from the experience. Treat yourself with kindness and understanding, and forgive yourself for any setbacks.

- Distract Yourself: divert your attention by doing something exciting or engaging when the need to emotionally eat comes. Go for a walk, listen to music, take a hot bath, or immerse yourself in a hobby to shift your focus away from food and reduce emotional distress.

- Professional Assistance: if you're having trouble reining in your emotional eating, you may want to consider seeking guidance from a certified therapist or counselor. Therapy can help you explore the underlying emotional triggers for your eating behavior and develop effective coping strategies to address them.

Addressing Plateaus and Setbacks

Plateaus and setbacks are common occurrences on the journey of intermittent fasting. They can be frustrating and demotivating, but they are also opportunities for growth and learning.A plateau occurs when progress appears to stall or plateau, despite consistent adherence to an intermittent fasting regimen. It can manifest in various ways, such as a lack of weight loss, decreased energy levels, or stagnation in fitness improvements. Setbacks, on the other hand, involve unexpected obstacles that disrupt progress, such as illness, injury, or periods of intense stress.

The Impact of Plateaus and Setbacks on Intermittent Fasting

Plateaus and setbacks can have a significant impact on morale and motivation, leading individuals to question the effectiveness of their fasting regimen or their ability to achieve their health goals. They may feel discouraged and tempted to abandon their fasting protocol altogether. However, it's essential to recognize that plateaus and setbacks are a natural part of any journey, and they do not signify failure.

Some of the impact of plateaus and setbacks include:

- Psychological Impact: Plateaus and setbacks can take a toll on an individual's mental well-being, leading to feelings of frustration, disappointment, and discouragement. Many individuals invest considerable time and effort into their fasting journey, and when progress stalls or obstacles arise, it can be disheartening. These feelings may contribute to a negative mindset, self-doubt, and a loss of motivation to continue with intermittent fasting.

- Stalled Progress: Plateaus often result in a lack of visible progress, whether it be in terms of weight loss, body composition changes, or improvements in health markers. Despite adhering to a fasting protocol, individuals may find that their efforts do not yield the desired results, leading to a sense of stagnation and a feeling of being stuck in a rut. Setbacks, such as illness or injury, can also disrupt progress and delay achieving health goals.

- Physical Effects: Plateaus and setbacks may have physical effects on the body, such as changes in metabolism, energy levels, and hormonal balance. Individuals may experience fluctuations in energy, mood swings, and changes in appetite, which can further complicate adherence to an intermittent fasting regimen. Additionally, prolonged plateaus may lead to feelings of fatigue and burnout, impacting overall well-being and quality of life.

- Deterioration of Habits: Plateaus and setbacks can undermine healthy habits and routines established during intermittent fasting. Individuals may be tempted to revert to old, unhealthy eating patterns or abandon their fasting protocol altogether in response to challenges or setbacks. This can perpetuate a cycle of yo-yo dieting, making it difficult to achieve sustainable results and maintain long-term success with intermittent fasting.
- Loss of Motivation: Plateaus and setbacks can sap motivation and enthusiasm for the fasting journey. When progress is slow or non-existent, individuals may question the efficacy of intermittent fasting and their ability to achieve their health goals. This loss of motivation can make it challenging to stay committed to fasting, leading to a lack of consistency and adherence to the protocol.
- Impact on Self-Confidence: Plateaus and setbacks can erode self-confidence and self-esteem, particularly if individuals perceive themselves as failing to meet their expectations or the expectations of others. These challenges may trigger feelings of inadequacy, self-doubt, and negative self-talk, which can undermine self-efficacy and belief

in one's ability to succeed with intermittent fasting.

- Social and Emotional Effects: Plateaus and setbacks can have social and emotional repercussions, affecting relationships and overall well-being. Individuals may feel isolated or misunderstood if friends or family members do not support their fasting journey or fail to recognize the challenges they face. Emotional eating or seeking comfort in food may also become more prevalent during times of frustration or stress, further complicating efforts to overcome plateaus and setbacks.

Practical Tips for Addressing Plateaus and Setbacks

Reassess Your Approach: If you've hit a plateau, it may be time to reassess your approach to intermittent fasting. Evaluate factors such as your fasting schedule, meal composition, calorie intake, and activity level to identify areas for improvement or modification.

1. Adjust Your Eating Window: Consider adjusting the length or timing of your eating window to see if it helps break through a plateau. Experiment with different fasting protocols, such as alternate-day fasting or time-restricted feeding, to find the approach that works best for your body.

2. Focus on Nutrient-Dense Foods: Pay attention to the quality of your food choices during your eating window. Emphasize nutrient-dense, whole foods such as fruits, vegetables, lean proteins, and healthy fats to support overall health and well-being.

3. Incorporate Regular Physical Activity: Regular exercise can help boost metabolism, increase energy expenditure, and support weight loss efforts. Incorporate a mix of cardiovascular exercise, strength training, and flexibility exercises into your routine to maximize results.

4. Stay Consistent: Consistency is key to overcoming plateaus and setbacks. Stick to your intermittent fasting schedule, even when progress seems slow or non-existent. Trust the process and remain committed to your goals.

5. Monitor Your Progress: Keep track of your progress using tools such as a food diary, weight log, or fitness tracker. Monitoring your results allows you to identify patterns, track changes over time, and make adjustments as needed.

6. Stay Hydrated: Drinking an adequate amount of water is essential for overall health and well-being, including during periods of fasting. Ensure you stay hydrated while fasting.

7. Manage Stress: Stress can impact hormone levels, appetite, and metabolism, potentially contributing to plateaus and setbacks. Incorporate stress management techniques such as meditation, deep breathing, yoga, or mindfulness practices to help reduce stress levels and support overall health.

8. Get Adequate Sleep: Quality sleep is crucial for overall health and well-being, including metabolism, appetite regulation, and hormone balance. Aim for seven to nine hours of quality sleep per night to support your intermittent fasting journey.

9. Seek Support: Don't hesitate to reach out for support from friends, family members, or online communities when facing plateaus or setbacks. Sharing your challenges and experiences with others can provide encouragement, accountability, and valuable insights.

Plateaus and setbacks are inevitable on the journey of intermittent fasting, but they do not have to derail your progress or diminish your success.

CHAPTER 6

INTERMITTENT FASTING AND HORMONAL HEALTH

Understanding the Impact of Intermittent Fasting on Hormones

Hormones are chemical messengers produced by the several glands that make up the endocrine system These hormones travel through the bloodstream and bind to specific receptors on target cells, where they regulate various physiological processes, including metabolism, growth and development, reproduction, and mood.

Some of the key hormones involved in metabolism and energy regulation include insulin, glucagon, cortisol, growth hormone, and leptin. These hormones play critical roles in regulating blood sugar levels, mobilizing energy stores, and maintaining metabolic homeostasis.

The Impact of Intermittent Fasting on Hormones

The hormonal response to fasting is a complex and intricately regulated process that involves multiple hormones working together to maintain energy balance, stabilize blood glucose levels, and support cellular function. Fasting triggers a series of hormonal changes in the body that help mobilize energy reserves, switch from glucose to fat metabolism, and promote cellular repair and renewal. Understanding the hormonal response to fasting is crucial for comprehending how intermittent fasting impacts various aspects of metabolism, appetite regulation, and overall health.

- Insulin:

Insulin is a hormone produced by the pancreas that plays a central role in regulating blood glucose levels. Its primary function is to facilitate the uptake of glucose into cells, where it can be used for energy or stored for future use. When blood glucose levels rise after a meal, insulin is released to help transport glucose into cells. However, during fasting, insulin levels decrease to allow the body to access stored energy reserves, such as glycogen and fat, for fuel.

- Glucagon:

The pancreas produces the hormone glucagon, which opposes the effects of insulin. It stimulates the breakdown of glycogen in the liver, releasing glucose into the bloodstream to maintain blood sugar levels during fasting. Glucagon levels rise in response to low blood glucose levels, signaling the liver to convert stored glycogen into glucose for use by the body.Intermittent fasting can increase glucagon levels, promoting the mobilization of stored energy reserves and supporting fat burning.

- Cortisol:

Cortisol is a stress hormone produced by the adrenal glands that plays a crucial role in metabolism, immune function, and stress responses. During fasting, cortisol levels may increase slightly to help mobilize energy reserves and support gluconeogenesis, the process by which the liver produces glucose from non-carbohydrate sources, such as amino acids and glycerol. Cortisol also helps regulate blood pressure and suppress inflammation during periods of fasting.

- Growth Hormone:

Growth hormone is secreted by the pituitary gland and plays a key role in growth, metabolism, and body composition. Fasting stimulates the release of growth hormone, which promotes fat metabolism, muscle preservation, and cellular repair and regeneration. Growth hormone levels increase during fasting to help preserve lean muscle mass and support metabolic adaptations to periods of energy restriction.

- Leptin:

The hormone leptin, which is generated by fat cells, aids in controlling hunger and energy balance. It signals to the brain when energy stores are sufficient, suppressing appetite and increasing energy expenditure. During fasting, leptin levels may decrease temporarily, leading to increased hunger and appetite as the body seeks to replenish energy reserves. However, long-term fasting can lead to adaptations in leptin sensitivity, helping to regulate appetite and energy balance over time.

- Adiponectin:

Adiponectin is a hormone secreted by fat cells that plays a role in regulating glucose and lipid metabolism. Fasting has been shown to increase adiponectin levels, which may contribute to improved insulin sensitivity, reduced inflammation, and enhanced fat burning. Higher levels of adiponectin are associated with a lower risk of metabolic disorders, such as type 2 diabetes and cardiovascular disease.

- Norepinephrine and Epinephrine:

Norepinephrine and epinephrine, also known as adrenaline, are hormones released by the adrenal glands in response to stress or danger. During fasting, levels of these hormones may increase to help mobilize energy reserves, increase metabolic rate, and support cognitive function. Norepinephrine and epinephrine play a role in promoting fat breakdown, increasing heart rate and blood pressure, and enhancing alertness and focus during fasting.

- Endorphins:

Endorphins are neurotransmitters produced by the brain that act as natural painkillers and mood enhancers. Fasting has been shown to increase endorphin levels, which may contribute to feelings of euphoria, well-being, and mental clarity. Endorphins help alleviate stress, reduce anxiety, and improve mood during fasting, making it easier to adhere to a fasting regimen and maintain motivation.

- Reproductive Hormones

Intermittent fasting may also impact reproductive hormones such as estrogen and progesterone, which play key roles in menstruation, fertility, and overall reproductive health in women. Some research suggests that intermittent fasting may alter menstrual cycles and hormone levels in women, although more studies are needed to fully understand these effects.

Potential Benefits of Hormonal Changes with Intermittent Fasting

While the hormonal changes induced by intermittent fasting may seem daunting, they can also confer several potential health benefits for women.

Improved insulin sensitivity, for example, can help reduce the risk of type 2 diabetes and metabolic syndrome.

Additionally, fluctuations in leptin and ghrelin levels may enhance appetite regulation and promote weight loss in women following an intermittent fasting regimen.

Intermittent fasting has anti-inflammatory effects, which may help reduce inflammation in the body and lower the risk of chronic diseases such as heart disease, cancer, and Alzheimer's disease. By reducing oxidative stress and inflammation, intermittent fasting supports overall health and longevity.

Some studies suggest that intermittent fasting may increase lifespan and promote longevity by activating cellular repair mechanisms and enhancing resilience to stress. By optimizing hormone levels and promoting cellular rejuvenation, intermittent fasting may help slow the aging process and extend lifespan.

Furthermore, some research suggests that intermittent fasting may have positive effects on hormone-related conditions such as polycystic ovary syndrome (PCOS) and menopausal symptoms, although more research is needed in these areas.

In conclusion, fasting elicits a coordinated hormonal response that helps the body adapt to periods of energy restriction and support metabolic flexibility.

Navigating Menopause, Perimenopause and Intermittent Fasting.

The normal biological process of menopause signifies the end of a woman's reproductive years. It typically occurs between the ages of 45 and 55, although the timing can vary widely among individuals.

Contrarily, the transitional stage before menopause is referred to as the perimenopause. The hormonal changes that occur during perimenopause and menopause are primarily driven by a decline in the production of estrogen and progesterone by the ovaries.

These hormonal fluctuations can have a wide range of effects on women's health, including changes in metabolism, bone density, cardiovascular health, cognitive function, and mood.

In recent years, intermittent fasting has gained attention as a potential strategy for managing symptoms associated with menopause and perimenopause, as well as promoting overall hormonal health in women, we'll look at how fasting can be used as a tool to navigate hormonal changes during this transitional phase of life.

Understanding Menopause and Perimenopause

Perimenopause:

Perimenopause, often referred to as the menopausal transition, typically begins several years before menopause and can last for an average of four to eight years. However, the duration can vary widely among women. Perimenopause is characterized by fluctuations in hormone levels, particularly estrogen and progesterone, which can result in irregular menstrual cycles and various physical and emotional symptoms.

Perimenopause usually begins in a woman's 40s, although it can start earlier or later for some women. The average age of onset is around 45 years old, but it can occur as early as the mid-30s or as late as the early 50s.

During perimenopause, the ovaries gradually produce less estrogen and progesterone, leading to changes in the menstrual cycle. Estrogen levels may fluctuate, causing irregular periods, shorter or longer cycles, and changes in menstrual flow. Progesterone levels may also decline, leading to symptoms such as breast tenderness and mood swings.

Common symptoms of perimenopause include hot flashes, night sweats, sleep disturbances, vaginal dryness, mood swings, irritability, fatigue, and changes in libido. From woman to woman, these symptoms might differ in intensity and length.

While fertility declines during perimenopause due to changes in hormone levels and ovarian function, it is still possible for women to become pregnant until they reach menopause. However, the likelihood of conception decreases as women approach menopause, and the risk of miscarriage and chromosomal abnormalities increases.

Menopause:

The menstrual cycle permanently ceasing to occur, symbolic of a woman's end of reproductive years, is known as the menopause. It occurs when the ovaries stop releasing eggs and producing estrogen and progesterone. Menopause is considered complete when a woman has gone without a menstrual period for 12 consecutive months.

The average age of menopause in women is around 51 years old. However, menopause can occur sooner or later for some women. Women who undergo surgical removal of the ovaries (oophorectomy) or certain cancer treatments may experience premature menopause.

During menopause, estrogen and progesterone levels decline significantly, leading to the cessation of ovulation and menstruation. As a result, women may experience a range of symptoms related to hormonal fluctuations, including hot flashes, night sweats, vaginal dryness, mood swings, and changes in libido.

In addition to the symptoms experienced during perimenopause, women may also experience long-term changes such as thinning hair, dry skin, weight gain, loss of breast fullness, and changes in body composition. These symptoms can vary in intensity and duration, with some women experiencing mild symptoms while others may experience more severe discomfort.

Menopause is associated with an increased risk of certain health conditions, including osteoporosis, heart disease, and cognitive decline. The decline in estrogen levels can contribute to bone loss and increased risk of fractures, as well as changes in cholesterol levels and blood pressure that can affect heart health. Additionally, hormonal changes during menopause may impact cognitive function and increase the risk of conditions such as Alzheimer's disease.

Navigating Menopause and Perimenopause

Navigating menopause and perimenopause requires a proactive approach to managing symptoms and maintaining overall health and well-being. While hormone replacement therapy (HRT) and other medications may be prescribed to alleviate symptoms, lifestyle factors such as diet, exercise, stress management, and sleep hygiene can also play a significant role in managing menopausal symptoms and reducing health risks.

Impact of Intermittent Fasting on Hormonal Health During Menopause and Perimenopause

Intermittent fasting has been shown to have several potential benefits for hormonal health during menopause and perimenopause. Let's explore some of these benefits:

- Improved Insulin Sensitivity: Insulin resistance and fluctuations in blood sugar levels are common during perimenopause and menopause, contributing to weight gain and an increased risk of type 2 diabetes. Intermittent fasting can help improve insulin sensitivity and regulate blood sugar levels by promoting the utilization of stored glucose for energy during fasting periods. This can help reduce the risk of insulin resistance and support metabolic health during menopause and perimenopause.

- Enhanced Weight Management: Weight gain is a common symptom of menopause and perimenopause, attributed in part to hormonal changes and metabolic shifts. Intermittent fasting may help women manage their weight during this transitional phase by promoting fat loss, preserving lean muscle mass, and regulating appetite and calorie intake. By creating a calorie deficit and promoting fat oxidation, intermittent fasting can support weight loss and weight maintenance in women experiencing menopausal weight gain.

- Regulation of Hormonal Balance: Intermittent fasting may help regulate hormonal balance during menopause and perimenopause by modulating levels of key hormones such as estrogen, progesterone, and insulin. Some research suggests that intermittent fasting may help reduce estrogen dominance, a common hormonal imbalance associated with menopausal symptoms such as hot flashes and mood swings. By promoting hormonal balance, intermittent fasting may alleviate symptoms of menopause and improve overall well-being in women.

- Reduction of Menopausal Symptoms: Hot flashes, night sweats, mood swings, and other menopausal symptoms can significantly impact a woman's quality of life during perimenopause and menopause. Intermittent fasting may help reduce the severity and frequency of these symptoms by modulating hormone levels, reducing inflammation, and improving metabolic function. Additionally, intermittent fasting has been shown to support brain health and cognitive function, which may help alleviate mood swings and cognitive symptoms associated with menopause.

- Protection Against Age-Related Diseases: Women are at increased risk of developing certain age-related diseases such as osteoporosis, cardiovascular disease, and cognitive decline during and after menopause. Intermittent fasting has been associated with a reduced risk of these diseases by promoting cardiovascular health, supporting bone density, and enhancing cognitive function. By reducing oxidative stress, inflammation, and insulin resistance, intermittent fasting may help mitigate the risk of age-related diseases and promote healthy aging in women during menopause and beyond.

CHAPTER 7

TIPS FOR BUSY WOMEN

Incorporating Intermittent Fasting into a Busy Lifestyle

In today's fast-paced world, finding time for self-care and healthy habits can be challenging, especially for busy women juggling multiple responsibilities. However, incorporating intermittent fasting into a busy lifestyle is not as daunting as it may seem. With some strategic planning and simple adjustments, intermittent fasting can become a seamless part of your daily routine, helping you revitalize your energy and improve your health.

1. **Plan Your Meals and Eating Windows**
- Take some time each week to plan your meals and eating windows. Choose nutrient-dense foods that will keep you satisfied and energized throughout the day.
  Consider preparing meals in advance and batch cooking on weekends to save time during the week. This way, you'll have healthy options readily available during your eating windows.

2. **Optimize Your Eating Window**

- Choose an eating window that aligns with your schedule and preferences. Some women find it easier to fast during the morning hours and eat their first meal later in the day, while others prefer to skip dinner.

  Experiment with different eating windows to find what works best for you. Remember that flexibility is key, so don't be afraid to adjust your eating window as needed to accommodate your lifestyle.

3. **Stay Hydrated During Fasting Periods**

- Drink plenty of water, herbal tea, and other non-caloric beverages during fasting periods to stay hydrated and curb hunger. Aim to drink at least 8-10 glasses of water per day to support overall health and well-being.

  Avoid sugary drinks and caffeinated beverages that may disrupt your fasting state and spike insulin levels. Stick to water, herbal tea, black coffee, and other low-calorie options instead.

4. **Listen to Your Body**:

- Pay attention to your body's hunger and fullness cues during fasting periods. If you're feeling lightheaded, fatigued, or overly hungry, it may be a sign that you need to adjust your fasting schedule or break your fast earlier.

Don't push yourself too hard or feel guilty if you need to break your fast early occasionally. Remember that intermittent fasting is meant to be a flexible and sustainable lifestyle approach, not a rigid diet plan.

5. **Stay Busy and Distracted:**
- Keep yourself occupied and distracted during fasting periods to take your mind off food. Engage in activities such as work, exercise, hobbies, or spending time with loved ones to pass the time and prevent boredom eating. Consider incorporating mindfulness techniques such as deep breathing, meditation, or yoga to help manage cravings and reduce stress during fasting periods.

6. **Be Prepared for Social Situations**:
- Plan ahead for social gatherings, events, and meals out to ensure that you can stick to your fasting schedule while still enjoying social interactions. Eat a satisfying meal before attending events to avoid temptation and make healthier choices when dining out. Don't be afraid to communicate your dietary preferences and fasting goals with friends, family, and colleagues. Most people will be supportive and accommodating once they understand your reasons for intermittent fasting.

7. **Prioritize Self-Care and Rest:**

- During your fasting times, keep in mind that self-care and relaxation are important . Getting enough sleep, managing stress, and practicing relaxation techniques are essential for overall health and well-being. Avoid overexerting yourself or engaging in intense exercise during fasting periods, as this can increase feelings of fatigue and hunger. Instead, focus on gentle movement, stretching, and low-impact activities to support your body's needs.

Quick and Easy Meal Ideas

In the hustle and bustle of everyday life, finding time to prepare healthy meals can often feel like a daunting task, especially for busy women over 40. However, with a bit of creativity and planning, it's possible to enjoy delicious and nutritious meals that are quick and easy to prepare, even while following an intermittent fasting regimen. Below are a variety of simple and convenient meal ideas that will help you stay on track with your intermittent fasting goals without sacrificing taste or nutrition.

- **Smoothies and Shakes:**

Smoothies are a convenient and versatile option for busy women on the go. Simply blend together your favorite fruits, vegetables, protein powder, and liquid base (such as almond milk or coconut water) for a quick and nutritious meal or snack.

To keep things interesting, try out various taste combinations and components. Try adding leafy greens like spinach or kale, healthy fats like avocado or nut butter, and superfoods like chia seeds or flaxseeds for an extra nutritional boost.

- **Salads and Grain Bowls:**

Salads and grain bowls are another easy and customizable option for busy women. Start with a base of leafy greens, whole grains (such as quinoa or brown rice), and lean protein (such as grilled chicken or tofu), then add your favorite veggies, nuts, seeds, and dressings.

Prep your ingredients in advance and store them in separate containers for easy assembly throughout the week. Mason jar salads are a convenient option for taking on the go.

- **Egg-Based Dishes**:

Eggs are a nutrient-dense and versatile ingredient that can be used in a variety of quick and easy meals. Whip up a veggie-packed omelet, frittata, or scramble for a protein-rich breakfast, lunch, or dinner option.

Hard-boiled eggs make for a convenient and portable snack that can be enjoyed on its own or added to salads, sandwiches, or grain bowls for extra protein and flavor.

- **One-Pot Meals:**
One-pot meals are a lifesaver for busy women looking to minimize cleanup and maximize convenience. Try recipes like stir-fries, soups, stews, and chili that can be cooked in a single pot or pan for quick and easy prep.
Batch cooking these meals in advance and portioning them out into individual servings can save even more time during the week. Store leftovers

in the fridge or freezer for grab-and-go meals whenever you need them.

- **Snack Plates:**

Snack plates are a fun and flexible option for busy women who prefer grazing throughout the day. Fill a plate or bento box with a variety of healthy snacks like sliced veggies, hummus, nuts, seeds, cheese, fruit, and whole grain crackers.

Mix and match different flavors and textures to create a satisfying and balanced snack plate that will keep you energized and satisfied between meals.

- **Wrap and Sandwiches:**

Wraps and sandwiches are classic go-to options for quick and easy meals. Fill whole grain wraps or bread with lean protein, veggies, and spreads like avocado or hummus for a satisfying and portable meal.

Opt for whole grain or gluten-free bread and wraps for added fiber and nutrients. To maintain interest, try out various fillings and taste combos.

- **Prepared Meals and Convenience Foods:**

While homemade meals are always the best option, there's no shame in relying on prepared meals and convenience foods from time to time, especially when time is tight. Look for healthy options like pre-cooked grilled chicken, pre-cut veggies, canned beans, and pre-packaged salads or soups.

Just be sure to read labels carefully and choose options that are low in added sugars, sodium, and unhealthy fats. Aim for whole, minimally processed foods whenever possible.

Here's a three-week meal plan incorporating these meal ideas.

Week 1:

Day 1:

Breakfast: Green smoothie (spinach, banana, almond milk, protein powder)

Lunch: Quinoa salad with mixed vegetables, grilled chicken, and balsamic vinaigrette

Dinner: brown rice and a veggie stir-fry with tofu

Day 2:

Breakfast: omelet of vegetables with feta cheese, tomatoes, and spinach,

Lunch: Turkey and avocado wrap with whole grain tortilla

Dinner: Lentil soup with side salad and whole grain bread

Day 3:

Breakfast: Berry protein smoothie (mixed berries, Greek yogurt, almond milk)

Lunch: Cucumber, cherry tomatoes, and lemon-tahini dressing atop a bed of chickpea salad

Dinner: One-pot chicken and vegetable curry with quinoa

Day 4:
Breakfast: Scrambled eggs with sautéed peppers, onions, and mushrooms
Lunch: Caprese salad with tomatoes, basil, balsamic sauce, and fresh mozzarella.
Dinner: Roasted sweet potatoes, steamed broccoli, and grilled salmon.
Day 5:
Breakfast: Greek yogurt parfait topped with mixed berries and granola
Lunch: Hummus and veggie sandwich on whole grain bread
Dinner: Vegetable and tofu stir-fry with brown rice noodles

Week 2:
Day 6:
Breakfast: Spinach and mushroom frittata
Lunch: Quinoa and black bean salad with corn, avocado, and lime dressing
Dinner: Turkey chili with mixed beans and side salad
Day 7:
Breakfast: Banana almond butter smoothie (banana, almond butter, almond milk)
Lunch: Grilled chicken Caesar wrap with romaine lettuce and Caesar dressing
Dinner: turkey meatballs and spaghetti squash with marinara sauce.
Day 8:

Breakfast: Cottage cheese and fruit bowl with sliced peaches and almonds

Lunch: Mediterranean chickpea salad with olives, feta cheese, and Greek dressing

Dinner: Veggie-packed minestrone soup with whole grain bread

Day 9:

Breakfast: Coconut milk, mixed fruit, and chia seed pudding

Lunch: Turkey and cranberry wrap with mixed greens

Dinner: Baked cod with lemon herb sauce, roasted vegetables and qu

Day 10:

Breakfast: Breakfast: Breakfast burrito with black peas, scrambled eggs and salsa

Week 3:

Day 11:

Breakfast: Blueberry protein smoothie (blueberries, protein powder, almond milk)

Lunch: Veggie and hummus wrap with whole grain tortilla

Dinner: Lentil and vegetable curry with quinoa

Day 12:

Breakfast: Spinach and tomato omelet with goat cheese

Lunch: Caprese salad with grilled chicken and balsamic glaze

Dinner: Grilled shrimp skewers with roasted sweet potatoes and green beans

Day 13:

Breakfast: Greek yogurt with honey and sliced almonds

Lunch: Quinoa tabbouleh salad with chickpeas, cucumber, and lemon dressing

Dinner: Vegetable stir-fry with tofu and brown rice noodles

Day 14:

Breakfast: Cottage cheese and pineapple parfait with granola

Lunch: sandwich made with turkey and avocado on whole grain bread.

Dinner: Butternut squash soup with mixed greens salad

Day 15:

Breakfast: Breakfast burrito bowl with scrambled eggs, black beans, avocado, and salsa

Lunch: Mediterranean quinoa salad with grilled chicken, olives, and feta cheese

Dinner: Baked salmon with roasted vegetables and quinoa pilaf

Please feel free to modify the menu to fit your dietary requirements and personal preferences.

Strategies for Dining Out while Fasting

Dining out can be both a social pleasure and a culinary adventure, but for women over 40 practicing intermittent fasting, it can sometimes feel like a daunting challenge. However, with the right strategies in place, you can enjoy dining out while staying committed to your fasting goals.

Research Restaurants in Advance:
Before heading out, take a few moments to research restaurants in your area that offer fasting-friendly options. Many restaurants now provide their menus online, allowing you to preview meal choices and plan accordingly.
Look for establishments that offer a variety of protein-rich dishes, salads, and vegetable-based entrees. Avoid places known for their extensive dessert menus or all-you-can-eat buffets, as these can be tempting pitfalls for those fasting.

Choose the Right Time to Dine:
Timing is key when dining out while fasting. Whenever possible, schedule your restaurant visits during your eating window to ensure you can enjoy a satisfying meal without breaking your fast prematurely.
If dining out falls outside your eating window, plan your meal strategically by having a nutritious snack

or light meal beforehand. This can help curb excessive hunger and prevent overindulging later on.

Opt for Protein and Fiber:

When perusing the menu, prioritize dishes that are high in protein and fiber. Protein-rich foods like lean meats, fish, tofu, and legumes can help keep you feeling full and satisfied, while fiber-rich options like vegetables and whole grains aid in digestion and promote satiety.

Aim to build your meal around these nutrient-dense choices, steering clear of dishes laden with refined carbohydrates and unhealthy fats.

Practice Portion Control:

Restaurant portions are often much larger than what you would typically eat at home, making it easy to overindulge. To avoid this, consider sharing a meal with a friend or ordering an appetizer or side dish instead of a full entree.

If you do order an entree, ask for a to-go box upfront and portion out half of your meal to enjoy later. This way, you can still savor your favorite dishes without overdoing it.

Stay Hydrated:

Hydration is essential, especially when fasting. Opt for water, sparkling water, or herbal tea to stay hydrated throughout your meal. Not only will this help quench your thirst, but it can also aid digestion and prevent overeating.

Limit your intake of sugary sodas, alcoholic beverages, and other calorie-laden drinks, as these can add unnecessary calories and disrupt your fasting efforts.

Be Mindful of Temptations:

Restaurants are filled with tempting treats and indulgent options, but that doesn't mean you have to give in to every craving. Practice mindfulness and stay focused on your goals by reminding yourself of the benefits of intermittent fasting.

If you find yourself tempted by certain menu items, take a moment to pause and assess whether indulging is worth it. Consider whether the short-term pleasure of eating that dessert or fried appetizer aligns with your long-term health and wellness goals.

Flexibility is Key:

Remember that intermittent fasting is a flexible lifestyle approach, not a rigid diet plan. If you veer off course during a restaurant meal, don't be too hard on yourself. Instead, view it as an opportunity to learn and grow, and get back on track with your fasting routine as soon as possible.

The occasional dining out experience shouldn't derail your progress or cause you undue stress. By practicing moderation and mindfulness, you can strike a balance between enjoying restaurant meals and staying committed to your health goals.

CHAPTER 8

SAFETY AND PRECAUTIONS

Consulting with Healthcare Professionals

Before initiating intermittent fasting, it's essential to recognize that individual health profiles vary widely. Age, existing medical conditions, medications, hormonal fluctuations, and lifestyle habits all influence the suitability of intermittent fasting. Consulting with healthcare professionals is critical to identify potential risks, address concerns, and tailor the fasting approach to your specific needs.

The Role of Healthcare Professionals:

Primary Care Physicians

Your primary care physician serves as the cornerstone of your healthcare team. They possess a comprehensive understanding of your medical history, current health status, and potential risk factors. Engage in open dialogue with your physician about your intention to begin intermittent fasting.

Your physician can conduct a thorough health assessment, including physical examinations and laboratory tests, to evaluate your readiness for intermittent fasting. They may also adjust medications or treatments to accommodate fasting practices safely.

Registered Dietitians or Nutritionists

Registered dietitians or nutritionists specialize in personalized dietary guidance. They assess your nutritional needs, preferences, and health goals to develop a fasting plan tailored to your requirements. Seek guidance from a dietitian to ensure adequate nutrient intake and meal planning during fasting periods.

A dietitian can offer practical strategies for managing hunger, optimizing meal composition, and maintaining nutritional balance while fasting. They may also address specific dietary concerns, such as food allergies or intolerances, to enhance fasting compliance and effectiveness.

Endocrinologists

Hormonal changes associated with aging, particularly during menopause, can influence metabolic function and overall health. Consulting with an endocrinologist can provide valuable insights into the interplay between intermittent fasting and hormonal balance.

Endocrinologists conduct specialized assessments, including hormone testing and metabolic evaluations, to evaluate your hormonal health. They can offer targeted interventions or hormone replacement therapies, if necessary, to support hormonal balance and mitigate potential risks associated with fasting.

Mental Health Professionals

Psychological factors, such as stress, emotional eating, and body image concerns, can impact your relationship with food and fasting. Seek support from a mental health professional, such as a psychologist or therapist, to address underlying emotional issues.

Mental health professionals offer strategies for managing psychological challenges associated with fasting, such as stress-reduction techniques, cognitive behavioral therapy, and mindfulness practices. They can also provide guidance on developing a positive body image and healthy eating behaviors.

Key Considerations for Consultation:

Comprehensive Health Assessment:

Provide your healthcare provider with detailed information about your medical history, including past illnesses, surgeries, medications, and family medical history. This information enables them to assess your suitability for intermittent fasting and identify any potential contraindications.

Transparent Communication:

Clearly communicate your health goals, motivations for intermittent fasting, and any concerns or questions you may have. Open dialogue fosters collaboration between you and your healthcare provider, ensuring that your fasting plan aligns with your individual needs and preferences.

Ongoing Monitoring and Follow-Up:

Schedule regular follow-up appointments with your healthcare provider to monitor your progress, address any issues or challenges, and make adjustments to your fasting plan as needed. Ongoing monitoring allows for early detection of any adverse effects and ensures that your fasting regimen remains safe and effective.

Pregnancy, Menopause, and Fasting

Understanding Pregnancy and Fasting:

Pregnancy is a transformative period characterized by significant physiological changes to support fetal development. While intermittent fasting may offer benefits for non-pregnant individuals, it's essential to prioritize the health and safety of both the mother and the baby during pregnancy.

Consultation with Healthcare Professionals:

Before considering intermittent fasting during pregnancy, consult with your obstetrician or healthcare provider to assess the suitability of fasting based on your individual health status, medical history, and pregnancy-related factors.

Healthcare professionals can provide personalized guidance and recommendations tailored to your specific needs and circumstances, ensuring that any dietary modifications align with the requirements of a healthy pregnancy.

Nutritional Adequacy:

Pregnancy is a time of increased nutrient demands to support fetal growth and development. Fasting may compromise nutrient intake, potentially leading to nutrient deficiencies that can negatively impact maternal and fetal health.

Focus on consuming a balanced and nutrient-dense diet that provides essential vitamins, minerals, protein, and calories to support optimal pregnancy outcomes. Emphasize whole foods, including fruits, vegetables, lean proteins, whole grains, and healthy fats, to meet your nutritional needs.

Hydration and Fluid Intake:

Adequate hydration is crucial during pregnancy to support maternal circulation, fetal development, and overall well-being. Fasting may increase the risk of dehydration, especially in the absence of fluid intake during fasting periods.

Drink plenty of water throughout the day, aiming for at least 8-10 glasses of water daily, or more as needed to maintain hydration. Limit caffeine and sugary beverages, opting for water, herbal teas, and other hydrating fluids instead.

Gestational Diabetes Risk:

Pregnant women are at risk of developing gestational diabetes, a condition characterized by high blood sugar levels during pregnancy. Fasting may affect blood sugar regulation, potentially exacerbating the risk of gestational diabetes.

Monitor blood sugar levels regularly and consult with your healthcare provider if you have concerns about blood sugar management during fasting.

Follow dietary recommendations and lifestyle modifications to minimize the risk of gestational diabetes and promote optimal pregnancy outcomes.

Navigating Menopause and Fasting:

Menopause marks the end of reproductive function and brings hormonal changes that can impact metabolism, weight management, and overall health. While intermittent fasting may offer benefits for women approaching or during menopause, certain considerations should be taken into account to ensure safety and effectiveness.

Hormonal Fluctuations:

Menopause is associated with hormonal fluctuations, including declines in estrogen and progesterone levels. These hormonal changes can influence metabolism, appetite regulation, and body composition, potentially affecting the response to fasting.

Pay attention to how fasting affects your hormonal balance and overall well-being during menopause. Consult with healthcare professionals, such as endocrinologists or gynecologists, for personalized guidance and support.

Bone Health:

Osteoporosis, a disorder marked by decreasing bone density and an increased risk of fracture, is more common in postmenopausal women. Ensure adequate intake of calcium, vitamin D, and other nutrients essential for bone health. Incorporate dairy products, leafy greens, fortified foods, and supplements as needed to support bone density and reduce the risk of osteoporosis.

Cardiovascular Health:
Menopausal women are at higher risk of cardiovascular disease due to hormonal changes and age-related factors. Intermittent fasting may offer cardiovascular benefits, such as improved lipid profiles and blood pressure control, but individual responses may vary.
Monitor cardiovascular risk factors, such as blood pressure, cholesterol levels, and weight, while fasting during menopause. Adopt heart-healthy lifestyle habits, including regular exercise, a balanced diet, and stress management techniques, to promote cardiovascular health and reduce the risk of heart disease.

CONCLUSION

Dear Reader,

As we come to the conclusion of our journey through "Intermittent Fasting 101 for Women Over 40: Revitalize Your Energy and Health," I want to express my deepest gratitude for joining me on this transformative adventure. Together, we've delved into the intricacies of intermittent fasting, exploring its profound impact on health, vitality, and well-being.

Throughout this book, we've traversed a vast landscape of knowledge, from understanding the fundamentals of intermittent fasting to unraveling its practical applications for women over 40. Each chapter has been a testament to your commitment to self-improvement, your thirst for knowledge, and your unwavering dedication to your health and happiness.

At its core, intermittent fasting is more than just a dietary regimen -it's a philosophy, a way of life. By embracing fasting as a holistic approach to nourishing your body, nurturing your mind, and revitalizing your energy, you've embarked on a journey of self-discovery and transformation.

Reflecting on the insights you've gained, it's clear that intermittent fasting offers far-reaching benefits beyond weight loss alone. From improving metabolic health to enhancing cognitive function, the impact of fasting extends to every aspect of your well-being. By aligning your eating habits with your body's natural rhythms, you've unlocked the key to lasting health and vitality.

But perhaps the most profound revelation of all is the recognition that your journey is unique to you. As you navigate the complexities of intermittent fasting, remember that there is no one-size-fits-all approach. What works for one person may not work for you, and that's okay. Embrace the process, experiment with different protocols, and listen to your body's cues. Trust yourself, and know that you have the wisdom and intuition to chart your own path towards optimal health.

As you reflect on your intermittent fasting journey, celebrate your successes, no matter how small. Whether it's resisting temptation during a social gathering, hitting a new personal best in your workouts, or simply feeling more energized and vibrant, each victory is a testament to your strength, resilience, and determination.Reflection allows you to celebrate your successes, learn from your mistakes, and identify areas for improvement. It keeps you inspired and dedicated to your goals. Other benefits include

Increased self-awareness: Reflecting on your experiences can help you gain a better understanding of your habits, preferences, and challenges.

Enhanced motivation: Celebrating your successes and acknowledging your progress can boost your motivation and keep you focused on your goals.

Improved problem-solving skills: Reflection allows you to identify areas where you may be struggling and develop strategies to overcome obstacles.

Greater resilience: By reflecting on your past experiences, you can build resilience and confidence in your ability to overcome Challenges.

Deeper satisfaction: Reflecting on your journey can bring a sense of satisfaction and fulfillment as you see how far you've come and how much you've achieved.

But amidst the triumphs, there may also be challenges and setbacks along the way. Perhaps you encounter social pressures that make it difficult to adhere to your fasting schedule, or you find yourself grappling with cravings and emotional eating habits. Remember that these obstacles are not failures they are opportunities for growth and learning. Lean into discomfort, cultivate self-compassion, and embrace the journey, knowing that every setback is a stepping stone towards greater self-awareness and empowerment.

In navigating the complexities of intermittent fasting, it's essential to prioritize self-care and well-being above all else. Listen to your body's signals, honor its needs, and recognize when it's time to seek support from healthcare professionals. Whether you're navigating pregnancy, menopause, or other hormonal transitions, trust that you have the resources and resilience to navigate these challenges with grace and resilience.

Looking towards the future, I encourage you to approach your intermittent fasting journey with curiosity, openness, and a spirit of adventure. Embrace the opportunity to explore new fasting protocols, experiment with different eating windows, and discover what works best for you. Remember that the journey is ongoing, and there is always room for growth, evolution, and self-discovery.

As you move forward, I invite you to cultivate a sense of gratitude for the journey you've undertaken and the progress you've made. Celebrate your victories, no matter how small, and honor the resilience and determination that have brought you this far. Remind yourself that you have boundless potential and that you can do everything you put your mind to.

In closing, I want to thank you once again for allowing me to be a part of your intermittent fasting journey. It has been an honor and a privilege to share these insights with you, and I am inspired by your courage, resilience, and unwavering commitment to your health and happiness. As you continue on your path towards greater well-being, may you be filled with joy, abundance, and radiant health.

With warmest regards,

Ava T. Hills.